THE COMPLETE
FATTY LIVER DIET
COOKBOOK

1500 Days of Quick & Easy Low-Fat Recipes to Deep Cleanse your Liver and Promote Vitality | No-Stress 28-Day Meal Plan Included

Lena Garrett

© Copyright 2024 by Lena Garrett - All rights reserved.

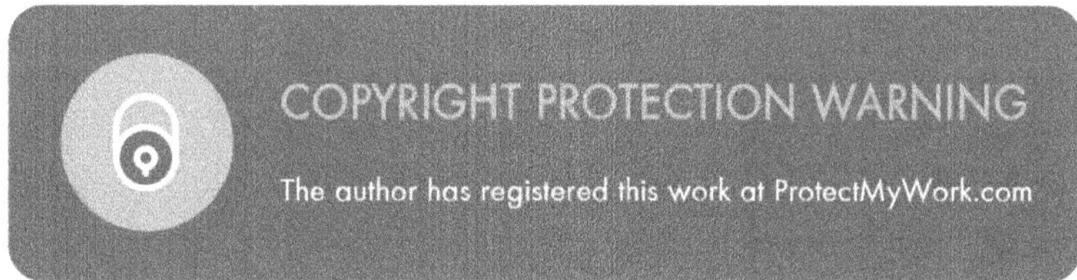

Table of Contents

INTRODUCTION

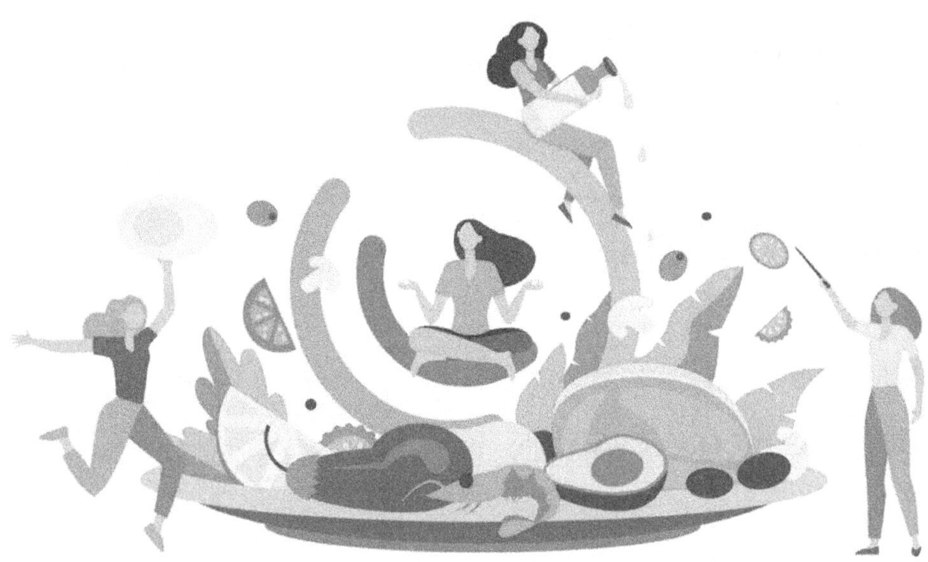

Understanding Fatty Liver Disease

Fatty liver disease is a condition where extra fat builds up in the liver. This organ is very important because it helps filter toxins out of your blood, makes substances that help your body work properly, and helps turn food into energy. When there's too much fat in the liver, however, these processes can be affected.

There are two main types of fatty liver disease: **alcohol-related** and **non-alcohol-related**. As you might guess, alcohol-related fatty liver disease (ARFLD) is due to heavy drinking over a long time. Non-alcohol-related fatty liver disease (NAFLD) isn't due to alcohol but often linked to being overweight or obese, having high blood sugar (often signaling pre-diabetes or actual diabetes) or high levels of fats in the blood.

So why does extra fat get stored in the liver? It could happen for several reasons. People who are obese or overweight might have bodies that send too much fat to the liver. If you eat more calories than you burn during physical activities, your body might convert these excess calories into fat and store it in the liver. This can also happen if you drink a lot of alcohol.

Now that we know what fatty liver disease is and what might cause it, we need to understand why it's a problem. Our body needs a healthy liver to survive. A fatty liver can become inflamed, which means it gets swollen and sensitive because of irritation or injury. This type of inflammation is called steatohepatitis and can lead to scarring known as fibrosis. If this scarring gets worse, it could lead to cirrhosis, where the liver shrinks and gets hard. If not caught early on, the damage could become so bad that you might need a new liver.

Besides cirrhosis, having fatty liver disease makes you more likely to develop health issues like heart problems, kidney disease, type 2 diabetes, and certain kinds of cancer. These complications are serious – they can seriously affect your quality of life and how long you live.

Understanding fatty liver disease helps us recognize the importance of eating well and staying active as part of taking care of our livers. It's not just about cutting out alcohol if you're drinking too much – it's also about managing what you eat and how much you move daily.

By being aware of this condition and its risks, we can take proactive steps toward maintaining a healthy diet rich in fruits, vegetables, lean proteins, and whole grains while also reducing high-calorie foods with lots of sugar or fat. Regular physical activity is equally essential; even walking more can make a difference.

Remember that knowledge is power in taking care of our health – by learning about fatty liver disease, its causes, and potential health risks, we're taking an important step in protecting our well-being.

How to Manage A Fatty Liver

Managing a fatty liver involves a blend of lifestyle adjustments and keen attention to your health. If you're facing the condition, also known as **hepatic steatosis**, take heart in knowing that it's manageable with the right steps.

1. **Lifestyle Modifications**: The cornerstone of managing a fatty liver is lifestyle change. Here are several key areas to focus on:

   a) *Healthy Weight:* Achieving and maintaining a healthy weight can reduce liver fat levels. Even a reduction of 10% in body weight can lead to significant improvements in liver health.

b) *Physical Activity:* Regular exercise helps burn triglycerides and decreases liver fat deposits. Aim for at least 150 mins of moderate-intensity activities like brisk walking or swimming each week.

c) *Alcohol Intake:* Minimize alcohol consumption as it can cause further liver damage. For AFLD, it's usually advised to avoid alcohol entirely.

2. **Medication Check**: Some drugs can exacerbate liver issues—consult with a healthcare provider about your current medications if you have a fatty liver.

3. **Monitor Your Health**: Routine checkups are necessary when managing fatty liver disease. This may involve:

a) Regular blood tests to check your liver enzyme levels.

b) Occasional ultrasounds or other imaging exams like CT scans or MRIs for visual tracking of the liver's condition.

4. **Control Comorbid Conditions**: Conditions like diabetes and high cholesterol can worsen fatty liver disease; managing these effectively is important:

a) If diabetic, maintaining blood sugar levels within the target range is crucial.

b) For high cholesterol, dietary changes along with prescribed medication might be needed to keep it under control.

5. **Avoid Certain Substances**: Toxins can stress the liver—limit exposure by:

a) Avoiding unnecessary medications or supplements.

b) Being cautious with chemicals, like those in cleaners and pesticides.

6. **Importance of Diet**: The food you eat plays a critical role in managing a fatty liver. Your diet should focus on reducing fat intake, especially saturated fats and trans fats, which can worsen liver fat accumulation. A detailed diet plan will come in the following chapters, but generally speaking:

a) Plenty of fruits, vegetables, whole grains, and healthy fats should be included.

b) Foods high in refined sugar and saturated fats should be limited.

c) Certain fish may be beneficial due to omega-3 fatty acids which support liver health.

7. **Stress Management**: Chronic stress may contribute to worsening a fatty liver situation due to hormonal changes that can affect your metabolism:

   a) Techniques such as deep breathing exercises, meditation, or yoga can help manage stress levels effectively.

8. **Stay Hydrated**: Water helps detoxify and maintain proper bodily functions including those of the liver; aim for at least eight glasses a day.

9. **Support Network**: Dealing with health conditions can be challenging; having friends or family as support or looking into support groups can make management easier mentally and emotionally.

Creating a structured plan that includes the above components is essential—consider mapping out daily routines that incorporate diet modifications, physical activities, physician appointments, and stress-relief strategies.

Purpose Of This Cookbook

Welcome to the **"Fatty Liver Diet Cookbook",** a guide designed not only to tantalize your taste buds but also to embark you on a journey toward better liver health. This cookbook serves a dual purpose: it is your companion in promoting a liver-friendly lifestyle while simultaneously balancing nutrition and flavor. Through these pages, you will discover that managing your liver health does not mean sacrificing delicious meals.

This book presents a carefully selected collection of recipes crafted specifically for those looking to improve or maintain their liver health without losing out on the joy of eating well-crafted dishes. Each recipe has been formulated with two key themes in mind: promoting a liver-friendly lifestyle and balancing nutrition with flavor.

Promoting a Liver-Friendly Lifestyle

A liver-friendly diet implies incorporating foods that are beneficial for maintaining healthy liver function and avoiding those which can contribute to its damage. By choosing ingredients that are high in fiber, low in saturated fats, and abundant in antioxidants, we pave the way toward enhancing the body's natural detox systems. It is all about making educated choices that favor whole grains, lean proteins, fruits, vegetables, and healthy fats found in nuts, seeds, and fishes rich in omega-3 fatty acids.

This cookbook equips you with recipes that include these powerful nutrients without requiring you to have advanced knowledge of nutrition. Each recipe provides straightforward instructions and simple ingredient lists that encourage even novice cooks to prepare meals beneficial for their livers. From energizing breakfast options to hearty dinners and light refreshments, you will find an assortment of meals adept at supporting your liver's health while fulfilling your dietary needs.

Balancing Nutrition and Flavor

All too often, diets focusing on health overlook the importance of flavor but not this one! With an understanding that satisfaction at the dining table is as crucial as nutritional content, we have been diligent in crafting recipes that deliver both. The flavorful profiles found within these pages have been thoroughly tested to ensure they are palatable while still adhering to the recommendations for preventing or managing fatty liver disease.

We combine herbs, spices, and seasonings from diverse culinary backgrounds to create delectable dishes that excite your palate without adding unnecessary calories or harmful ingredients. From zesty salads and tangy dressings to savory stews and sweet desserts made with natural sweeteners like honey or maple syrup each meal is an adventure for your taste buds!

This cookbook is an embodiment of our commitment to improving liver health through proper nutrition while upholding the pleasure derived from eating well-prepared food. It is meant for anyone who seeks not only to take care of their body but also enjoy every bite along their journey towards wellness.

As you turn each page and try new recipes from this book, remind yourself of the change you're making not just in your eating habits but also in your overall lifestyle. With each step forward on this path lined with wholesome ingredients seasoned by zestful flavors you're taking another step toward reclaiming your liver health. Let this cookbook be the first of many supports along your way to vitality!

CHAPTER 1: ESSENTIALS OF THE FATTY LIVER DIET

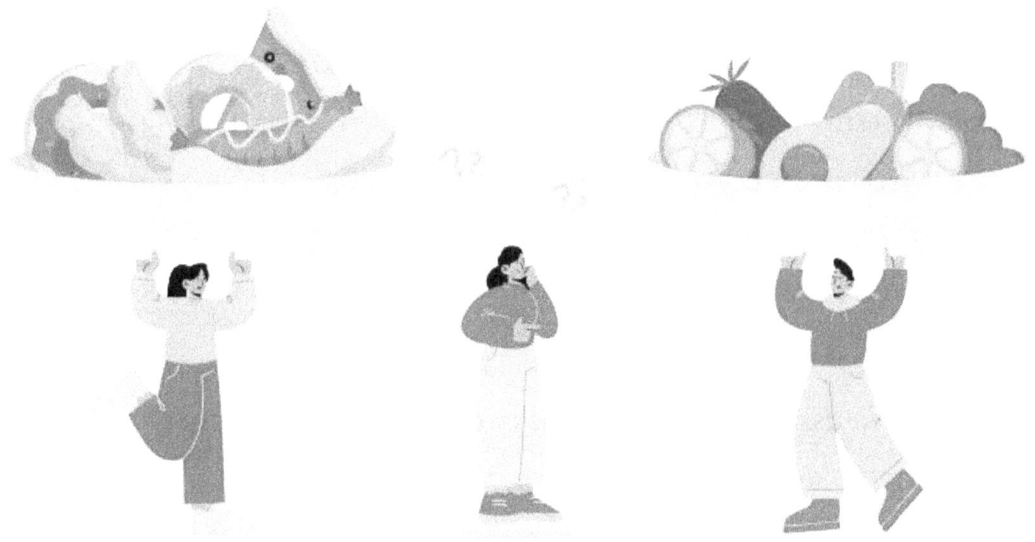

The liver is a powerhouse of an organ, fulfilling essential roles such as detoxification, protein synthesis, and chemical production for digestion. Unfortunately, it can fall victim to an unhealthy accumulation of fat, a condition known as fatty liver. In response to this growing health concern, the fatty liver diet has emerged as a beacon of hope for those seeking to restore their liver health through nutrition.

The **fatty liver diet** is a carefully curated eating plan aimed at reducing excess fat stored in the liver cells. It isn't just one specific diet; rather, it's a combination of eating patterns that emphasize whole foods, high fiber intake, and balanced macronutrients. This diet particularly limits items high in added sugars and saturated fats, as these can exacerbate liver fat accumulation.

Adopting a fatty liver diet has numerous benefits for overall health and particularly for enhancing liver function:

1. **Weight Management:** Losing weight can help reduce the amount of fat in your liver. For overweight individuals, even modest weight loss can make a significant difference in improving liver health.

2. **Improved Insulin Sensitivity:** A diet rich in fiber and low in refined sugars can increase the body's sensitivity to insulin, helping manage blood sugar levels more effectively.

3. **Decreased Inflammation:** Foods high in antioxidants and healthy fats can reduce inflammation not just in the liver but throughout the entire body.

4. **Enhanced Digestive Health:** High-fiber foods support a healthy digestive system by promoting bowel regularity and beneficial gut bacteria.

5. **Better Blood Lipid Profile:** Reducing intake of unhealthy fats and incorporating heart-healthy fats can improve cholesterol levels and lower the risk of heart disease.

When and how to start? The best time to start the fatty liver diet is as soon as you're aware that your liver health is at risk or if you've been diagnosed with fatty liver disease. It's important to begin gradually by making simple changes to your current diet:

1. Swap processed foods with whole-food alternatives like fruits, vegetables, whole grains, nuts, seeds, lean meats, fish, and legumes.

2. Reduce sugar intake by avoiding sweets and sugary beverages; opt for water or herbal teas instead.

3. Choose healthier fats like those found in avocados, olive oil, nuts, and seeds rather than butter or fried foods.

4. Increase fiber through vegetables, whole grains, and legumes.

5. Eliminate alcohol consumption entirely if possible since alcohol is a toxin that the liver must work hard to break down.

6. Plan your meals regularly and be mindful of portion sizes.

Embracing the principles of the fatty liver diet means making lasting lifestyle changes — this isn't just a quick fix but a new way of eating that should be sustainable over the long term. It's important to listen to your body's signals and adapt accordingly while remaining consistent with healthy choices.

Food Groups to Focus On

When managing a fatty liver condition, your diet plays a critical role in your health. Incorporating certain food groups can help protect your liver, reduce fat accumulation, and encourage overall well-being. Here are some beneficial foods to focus on:

1. **Fruits and Vegetables:** These are packed with vitamins, minerals, antioxidants, and fiber that aid in digestion and can help reduce liver inflammation. Opt for a colorful variety such as leafy greens, berries, oranges, and carrots.
2. **Whole Grains:** Rich in fiber, whole grains like brown rice, oats, barley, and whole-wheat products help maintain a healthy weight and reduce fat build-up in the liver.
3. **Lean Proteins:** Incorporate lean cuts of meat such as chicken breast, turkey, and fish. Plant-based proteins like lentils, chickpeas, and tofu are also excellent choices as they lack the saturated fats found in red meats.
4. **Healthy Fats:** Not all fats are bad! Include sources of monounsaturated and polyunsaturated fats like olive oil, avocados, nuts, and seeds which can help maintain healthy liver function.
5. **Low-Fat Dairy:** Choose low-fat options such as skim milk, yogurt without added sugars, and soft cheeses to fulfill your calcium requirements without overloading your liver with fats.

Foods to Limit or Avoid

Certain foods can exacerbate fatty liver disease by contributing to fat build-up or adding stress to hepatic processes. It's vital to limit or avoid these:

1. **Alcohol:** Alcohol is a direct toxin to the liver and can cause significant damage when consumed in excess. Those with fatty liver disease should eliminate or dramatically reduce alcohol intake.
2. **Sugary Foods:** Foods high in added sugars like soda, candy, pastries, and some cereals contribute to fat accumulation in the liver.
3. **Trans Fats:** Often found in processed foods like cakes, pie crusts, biscuits, frozen pizzas, cookies, crackers and most fried foods; trans fats should be avoided altogether.
4. **Refined Carbohydrates:** White bread, pasta made from white flour and other processed carbs can spike blood sugar levels which may lead to increased fat storage in the liver.

5. **Red Meat:** High consumption of red meat which is rich in saturated fat should be limited; opt for leaner proteins instead.

6. **Salt-Heavy Foods:** Excessive salt can lead to water retention and increased blood pressure; it is best to minimize intake of high-sodium items such as canned soups or vegetables, packaged snacks or meals.

It's not only about what you eat but also how you eat. Eating smaller portions spread throughout the day rather than big meals can help manage your weight better and thus aid your liver. Below is a simple chart summarizing dietary recommendations for those with fatty liver disease:

FOOD GROUP	EXAMPLES	RECOMMENDED ACTION
Fruits & Vegetables	Berries, Oranges, Leafy Greens	Include a variety
Whole Grains	Brown Rice, Oats	Incorporate regularly
Lean Proteins	Chicken Breast, Lentils	Choose over red meats
Healthy Fats	Olive Oil, Nuts	Use in moderation
Low-Fat Dairy	Skim Milk, Yogurt	Opt for low-fat options
Alcohol	Beer, Wine	Eliminate/Reduce markedly
Sugary Foods	Soda, Pastries	Avoid or limit strictly
Trans Fats	Fried Foods, Cookies	Eliminate completely
Refined Carbohydrates	White Bread, Pasta made from white flour	Reduce significantly
Red Meat	Beef, Pork	Limit consumption
Salt-Heavy Foods	Canned Soups, Packaged Snacks	Minimize intake

The food recommendations provided are geared toward creating a balanced diet that supports liver health and prevents further fat accumulation. It's essential to tailor these guidelines to fit individual nutritional needs and consult with a healthcare provider for personalized advice.

Reading Nutrition Labels

Understanding nutrition labels is crucial when managing a fatty liver diet. These labels are your key to identifying what is truly in the food you eat. Sugar and fat can go by many names, making them tricky to spot. The first step to identifying these hidden components in your food is to read the ingredient list carefully. Sugars may be listed as high fructose corn syrup, cane sugar, invert sugar, maltose, dextrose, or even fruit juice concentrates, among others.

Similarly, fats can be disguised under terms like hydrogenated oils, trans fats, and saturated fat. These types of fats are particularly harmful for those with fatty liver disease and should be limited as much as possible. To help you better identify these hidden sugars and fats, here's a basic chart:

HIDDEN SUGAR	HIDDEN FAT
High fructose corn syrup	Hydrogenated oils
Cane sugar	Saturated fat
Invert sugar	Trans fat
Maltose	
Dextrose	
Fruit juice concentrates	

When reading labels, also pay attention to the order in which ingredients are listed. Ingredients are listed by quantity from highest to lowest. This means if sugar or fat sources are at the top of the list, the product is likely high in these components.

The next crucial element of reading nutrition labels is understanding **serving sizes**. Labels will show the amount of calories and nutrients per serving, but this can be misleading if one doesn't realize how small a "serving" actually is.

Always compare the serving size on the package to the amount you actually consume. For example, if a bag of chips lists the nutrients for 10 chips and you have eaten 30 chips, you should multiply the nutritional information by three to understand how much you have actually ingested.

Keep in mind that packaged foods often contain more than one serving per package; if you eat the whole package without realizing it contains multiple servings, you might consume an excessive amount of sugar or fat without knowing it.

Let's look at an illustration to make this concept clearer:

Nutrition Facts (example product)

Serving size: *10 chips (28g)*

Serving Per Container: About 5

Amount Per Serving: *Calories: 150; Total Fat: 9g (Saturated Fat: 1.5g | Trans Fat: 0g); Cholesterol: 0mg; Sodium: 90mg; Total Carbohydrate: 16g (Dietary Fiber: 1g | Sugars: 2g)*

If someone consumes half of this bag (about 2.5 servings), they technically ingest:

(150 cal x 2.5 servings) = 375 calories,

(9g total fat x2.5 servings) = 22.5 grams of total fat...and so forth.

Reading nutrition labels isn't just about understanding what's on the label—it's about translating that information into your daily habits.

CHAPTER 2: TIPS FOR STAYING MOTIVATED AND ON-TRACK

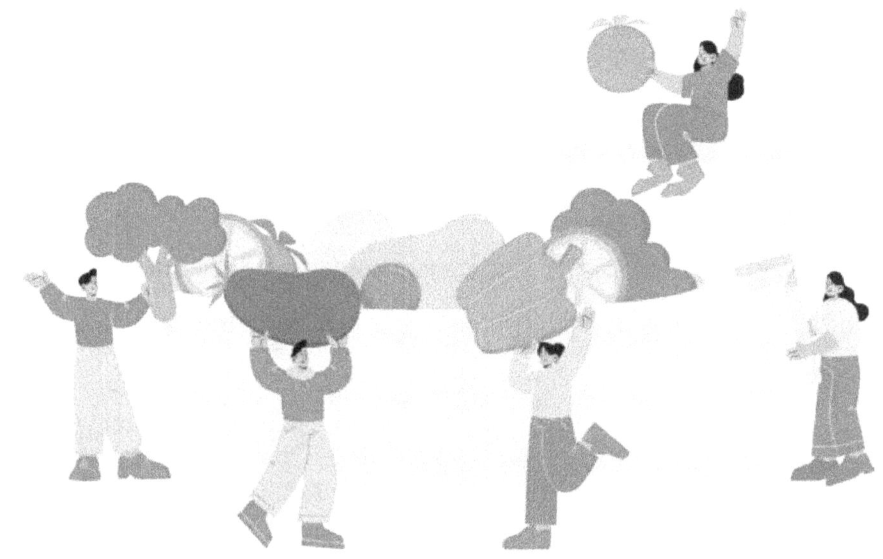

Connecting with Support Groups

When you're making dietary changes to manage a fatty liver, surrounding yourself with a supportive community can make all the difference. Support groups offer encouragement, accountability, and valuable insights from people who are facing similar challenges.

1. **Engagement:** Actively participate in support group meetings, whether online or in person. Being involved increases your sense of commitment and helps maintain your focus on health goals.

2. **Knowledge Sharing:** Use these groups as a knowledge base to learn from others' experiences. Discover new recipes, tips for managing cravings, and ways to integrate exercise into your routine that have worked for others.

3. **Encouragement:** Lean on the group during difficult times. If you're feeling demotivated or you've hit a plateau, chances are someone else has been there before and can offer advice.

4. **Celebrate Successes:** Share your own successes and celebrate those of others. Positive reinforcement is a powerful motivator.

Dealing with Setbacks

Setbacks are an inevitable part of any journey towards better health. Instead of viewing them as failures, consider them as learning opportunities that can foster resilience.

1. **Redefine Failure:** Understand that setbacks are not the end; they're simply part of the process. Remind yourself why you started this journey and the benefits you've already experienced.
2. **Small Steps:** Re-focus by setting small achievable targets instead of overwhelming yourself with bigr goals right away.
3. **Reflection:** Analyze what led to the setback without judgment. Identify triggers that may lead to unhealthy eating or skipping exercise and develop strategies to avoid them in the future.
4. **Self-compassion:** Be kind to yourself in the face of challenges. Self-criticism can be demoralizing while self-compassion can help boost your resolve to get back on track.

Prepping for Success

In addition to finding community support and dealing setbacks, personal preparation is key to maintaining your motivation. By setting clear, achievable goals, you create a roadmap for success that can guide you through tough moments.

Set SMART goals – Specific, Measurable, Achievable, Relevant, and Time-bound. When it comes to managing fatty liver through diet, your goals might include sticking to a meal plan, introducing more greens into your meals twice a week, or reducing processed sugars gradually till they are entirely out of your diet in two months. Here's a simple table to help organize your goals:

GOAL	ACTION ITEM	DEADLINE
Stick to meal plan	Prepare weekly meals in advance	Ongoing
Increase leafy greens	Add spinach to two meals per week	1 Month
Cut out processed sugar	Reduce daily sugar intake by 5g	2 Months

Remember that small steps add up over time; every small change contributes to a bigr transformation in managing your health.

Preparation goes beyond goal setting; it's also practical. Preparing meals ahead of time ensures that even when tiredness or temptation hits, you have healthy options readily available. Dedicate time each week to plan out meals—this includes shopping for ingredients as well as cooking. Eating out can be one of the biggest challenges when following a new diet plan. By having ready-to-eat meals or snacks at home or on-the-go, you resist the convenience of less healthy options.

Visual aids like charts tracking progress or inspirational messages placed where you will see them daily serve as powerful motivators. A photo on the refrigerator of what you hope to achieve or a chart marking off achieved milestones reminds you why you started this journey.

Recognizing achievements—no matter how small—is crucial for sustaining motivation. Treating yourself to something enjoyable (outside of food rewards) when reaching milestones helps solidify the positive association between hard work and positive outcomes.

CHAPTER 1. LIFESTYLE CHANGES TO SUPPORT YOUR DIET

Importance Of Exercise in Managing Fatty Liver

Exercise is not just beneficial for your waistline and heart; it also plays a crucial role in managing fatty liver. Engaging in physical activity can have a significant impact on reducing fat stored in the liver, thus improving liver function and overall health.

In individuals with fatty liver disease, regular exercise helps to improve insulin sensitivity. This is key because insulin resistance is often a precursor to fat accumulation in the liver, which can lead to non-alcoholic fatty liver disease (NAFLD). By enhancing the body's response to insulin, exercise helps keep blood sugar levels stable and prevents excess glucose from being converted into fat and deposited in the liver.

Moreover, exercise directly influences liver fat content. It stimulates the enzymes responsible for burning fat, leading to reduced fat storage. Even without weight loss, engaging in consistent physical activity can lead to significant reductions in visceral fat and intrahepatic lipid levels—the technical term for fat within your liver cells.

Studies have shown that both aerobic and resistance training are effective in managing fatty liver. **Aerobic exercise** like walking, cycling, or swimming increases heart rate and breathing, boosting overall calories burned and helping reduce liver fat. On the other hand, **resistance training** such as weight lifting improves muscle mass. Since muscle is a more metabolically active tissue than fat, having more muscle mass means your body will burn more calories at rest—aiding in the reduction of liver fat.

The American Heart Association recommends at least 150 mins per week of moderate-intensity aerobic activity or 75 mins per week of vigorous-intensity aerobic activity. However, it's important to remember that any amount of exercise is better than none. For those who are new to exercising or have limited mobility due to overweight or obesity commonly associated with fatty liver disease, low-impact activities like walking or stationary cycling are a great way to get started. For practical application, here's a simple weekly exercise chart that you can use as a starting point:

DAY	ACTIVITY	DURATION	INTENSITY
MON	Brisk Walking	30 mins	Moderate
TUE	Resistance Training	20 mins	Moderate-High
WED	Swimming	30 mins	Moderate
THU	Rest/Stretching	-	-
FRI	Cycling	30 mins	Moderate
SAT	Resistance Training	20 mins	Moderate-High
SUN	Recreational Sport	30 mins	Variable

It is always recommended to start slow and gradually increase both intensity and duration as your endurance improves. Also, it's crucial to check with your healthcare provider before beginning any new workout regimen—particularly if you have underlying health conditions related to your fatty liver diagnoses such as diabetes or cardiovascular disease.

Aside from directly reducing liver fat through improved metabolism and increased insulin sensitivity, exercise could also alleviate other aspects connected to NAFLD such as obesity, hypertension, cholesterol levels, all of which often go hand-in-hand with the condition.

Stress Reduction Techniques

Managing stress is a critical component of maintaining a healthy liver. Persistent stress can aggravate inflammatory processes, leading to increased fat accumulation in the liver, exacerbating conditions like fatty liver disease. Incorporating stress reduction techniques into your daily regimen can provide significant benefits for overall health and improve liver function.

1. Deep Breathing: Engaging in deep breathing exercises is a quick way to reduce stress. Here's a simple method:

> ➤ Find a quiet spot and sit or lie down comfortably.

- ➢ Place one hand on your chest and the other on your belly.
- ➢ Inhale slowly through your nose, feeling your belly rise, for four seconds.
- ➢ Hold your breath for another four seconds (if comfortable).
- ➢ Exhale slowly through your mouth, feeling the belly fall, over six seconds.
- ➢ Repeat this cycle for a few mins.

2. Progressive Muscle Relaxation: PMR involves tensing and then relaxing different muscle groups:

- ➢ Find a comfortable position and close your eyes.
- ➢ Start by tensing muscles in your feet for five seconds, then relax for 30 seconds.
- ➢ Gradually work up through each muscle group – legs, abdomen, chest, arms, neck, and face.
- ➢ Spend five seconds tensing each muscle group followed by 30 seconds of relaxation.

3. Mindful Eating: Eating should not just be about diet; how you eat is important too:

- ➢ Before eating, take a few deep breaths to center yourself.
- ➢ Eat slowly and without distractions like TV or smartphones.
- ➢ Pay attention to the taste, texture, and smell of your food.
- ➢ Listen to your body's hunger cues and stop eating when you're satisfied.

5. Yoga and Meditation: Both yoga and meditation can help relax the mind and body:

- ➢ Join a class or follow an online session designed for beginners.
- ➢ Try to practice yoga or meditate for at least 10-20 mins daily.

6. Adequate Sleep: Ensure you're getting enough sleep:

- ➢ Aim for 7-9 hours of quality sleep each night.
- ➢ Develop a regular sleep routine go to bed at the same time every night even on weekends.
- ➢ Avoid caffeine or heavy meals close to bedtime.

Incorporate these techniques into your daily routine to help manage stress levels effectively as part of your approach to treating fatty liver disease through diet and lifestyle changes.

Sleep Hygiene and Its Role in Liver Health

Sleep hygiene refers to the practices that contribute to quality and consistent sleep. Lack of sleep or disrupted sleep patterns can lead to increased stress on the body, including the liver. During sleep, the body undergoes various processes that are essential for liver function.

Sleep promotes the natural regeneration process of the liver. Just like our brains need sleep to process information, our livers need rest to process toxins. When we're asleep, our bodies enter a phase of restoration. For people with a fatty liver or other liver conditions, giving the organ time to repair and rejuvenate overnight is crucial for maintaining health.

Adequate sleep regulates metabolism. The liver plays a vital role in breaking down fats and converting them into usable energy. When we deprive ourselves of sleep, our metabolism can become sluggish, leading to less efficient fat processing by the liver a concern particularly relevant for those with fatty liver disease.

Sleep assists in hormonal balance. Hormones such as insulin are regulated during sleep which directly affects how the liver processes glucose and produces glucose stores known as glycogen. Proper glycogen storage in the liver is essential for overall metabolic health.

Good sleep reduces stress on the body and inflammation in the liver. Poor sleeping habits can increase stress hormones like cortisol which is harmful to liver cells over time and could exacerbate issues like inflammation a factor involved in many liver diseases.

Incorporating healthy sleep hygiene practices into one's routine can be beneficial for liver health:

1. **Maintain a consistent sleep schedule:** Go to bed and wake up at the same time every day.
2. **Create a restful environment:** Keep your bedroom dark, quiet, and cool.
3. **Avoid stimulants:** Cut down on caffeine and nicotine, especially in the hours leading up to bedtime.
4. **Exercise regularly:** But avoid vigorous activity close to bedtime.
5. **Limit screen time:** Reduce exposure to phones or computers before sleeping.
6. **Relaxation techniques:** Engage in activities such as reading or taking a bath before bed.

Adopting these simple yet effective bedtime rituals is an attainable goal we can all strive for to support our livers' long-term health. To reinforce why these steps matter specifically for those with fatty liver disease: The condition means there's an excessive amount of fat stored in the cells of the liver.

With proper rest helping manage weight, controlling blood sugar levels through hormone balance during sleep, and ensuring regular cleansing cycles by sticking to a consistent sleeping pattern – it's apparent how integral good sleep hygiene practices are in treating fatty liver disease.

CHAPTER 2. BREAKFAST RECIPES

1. Avocado and Spinach Smoothie Bowl

Preparation time: Ten mins

Cooking time: N/A

Servings: Two

Ingredients:

- One ripe avocado, peeled & pit removed
- Two cups fresh spinach leaves
- One cup unsweetened almond milk
- One tbsp chia seeds
- One tsp vanilla extract
- Half a cup of ice cubes

Directions:

1. In your blender, mix avocado, spinach, almond milk, chia seeds, vanilla extract, and ice cubes.
2. Blend on high speed till smooth. Serve.

Tips: For added texture, top with sliced almonds or hemp seeds before serving.

Serving size: 1 cup

Nutritional values (per serving): Calories: 234; Fat: 18g; Carbs: 15g; Protein: 4g; Sodium: 91mg; Sugar: 1g; Fiber: 9g

2. Kale and Turkey Breakfast Hash

Preparation time: Fifteen mins

Cooking time: Twenty mins

Servings: Four

Ingredients:

- Two tbsp olive oil
- Half a lb. lean ground turkey
- One big sweet potato, peeled and diced into half-inch pieces (approx. two cups)
- Four cups chopped kale leaves
- One tsp smoked paprika
- Half tsp powdered garlic
- Salt & pepper, as required

Directions:

1. Warm up one tbsp oil in your big non-stick skillet on moderate temp. Add ground turkey, then cook till browned, breaking it up. Remove turkey, then put aside.
2. In the same skillet, add the remaining oil along with diced sweet potatoes. Cook for ten mins till tender. Add kale, then sauté till wilted.
3. Add cooked turkey, then sprinkle with paprika, powdered garlic, salt, and pepper. Stir everything together and cook for another five mins.

Tips: To avoid added sugars or preservatives, choose fresh or dried spices over pre-mixed seasoning blends. You can substitute sweet potato with butternut squash for variety.

Serving size: One quarter of the recipe

Nutritional values (per serving): Calories: 256; Fat: 11g; Carbs: 20g; Protein: 17g; Sodium: 72mg; Sugar: 4g; Fiber: 3g

3. Chia Seed and Almond Pudding

Preparation time: Ten mins + chilling time

Cooking time: N/A

Servings: Two

Ingredients:

- Quarter cup of chia seeds

- One cup unsweetened almond milk

- One tbsp honey, optional

- Half tsp vanilla extract

- One tbsp sliced almonds

Directions:

1. In your container, mix chia seeds, almond milk, honey (if using), and vanilla extract. Cover, then put in refrigerator overnight till it thickens.

2. Stir the pudding once it's set to break up any clumps. Top with sliced almonds before serving.

Tips: For added texture, top with fresh berries or a sprinkle of cinnamon.

Serving size: Half of the total recipe

Nutritional values (per serving): Calories 180; Fat 9g; Carbs 20g; Protein 6g; Sodium 90mg; Sugar 9g; Fiber 10g

4. Herbed Chicken Sausage Patties

Preparation time: Ten mins

Cooking time: Fifteen mins

Servings: Four

Ingredients:

- One lb. ground chicken breast

- Two tbsp chopped fresh parsley

- One tbsp chopped fresh sage

- One tsp powdered garlic

- One tsp powdered onion

- Half tsp salt

- Quarter tsp black pepper

Directions:

1. In your big container, mix ground chicken, parsley, sage, powdered garlic, powdered onion, salt, and pepper. Form the mixture into eight patties.
2. Heat a non-stick skillet on moderate temp. Cook the patties for seven to eight mins per side till golden brown.

Tips: Use gloves or slightly wet hands to form patties to prevent sticking.

Serving size: Two patties

Nutritional values (per serving): Calories: 150; Fat: 3g; Carbs: 1g; Protein: 26g; Sodium: 450mg; Sugar: 0g; Fiber: 0g

5. Tofu Scramble with Mixed Peppers

Preparation time: Ten mins

Cooking time: Fifteen mins

Servings: Two

Ingredients:

- One lb. firm tofu
- One cup mixed bell peppers, diced
- Two tbsp nutritional yeast
- Half tsp turmeric
- One tbsp olive oil
- Quarter tsp black pepper
- Half tsp salt (optional)

Directions:

1. Press tofu for ten mins to remove excess moisture. Crumble into bite-sized pieces.
2. Heat olive oil in a skillet on moderate-high temp. Add the crumbled tofu and turmeric, stirring to combine.
3. Cook for five mins, then add the mixed bell peppers, then flavor it with nutritional yeast, black pepper, and salt if desired.

4. Stir well and cook for an additional ten mins or till peppers are soft and the tofu is lightly browned.

Tips: Pressing the tofu is crucial for texture; using non-stick cookware can reduce the need for oil.

Serving size: Half of the total recipe

Nutritional values (per serving): Calories: 150; Fat: 9g; Carbs: 8g; Protein: 14g; Sodium: 330mg; Sugar: 3g; Fiber: 4g

6. Low-Fat Greek Yogurt with Nuts and Honey

Preparation time: Five mins

Cooking time: N/A

Servings: Two

Ingredients:

- One cup low-fat Greek yogurt
- Two tbsp mixed nuts, chopped (such as almonds and walnuts)
- One tbsp honey
- Quarter tsp cinnamon (optional)

Directions:

1. Spoon half a cup of Greek yogurt into each bowl. Sprinkle one tbsp of chopped nuts over each serving of yogurt.
2. Drizzle half a tbsp of honey on top of each serving and add a dash of cinnamon if desired.

Tips: Choosing unsalted nuts will keep the sodium content low, which is better for a fatty liver diet.

Serving size: Half of the total recipe

Nutritional values (per serving): Calories: 180; Fat: 8g; Carbs: 18g; Protein: 10g; Sodium: 45mg; Sugar: 15g; Fiber: 1g

7. Sugar-Free Spirulina Protein Shake

Preparation time: Five mins

Cooking time: N/A

Servings: Two

Ingredients:

- Two cups unsweetened almond milk
- One tbsp spirulina powder
- One cup spinach leaves, fresh
- Half cup Greek yogurt, plain and low-fat
- One tbsp chia seeds
- One tsp vanilla extract
- Six ice cubes

Directions:

1. In your blender, mix almond milk, spirulina powder, fresh spinach leaves, Greek yogurt, chia seeds, vanilla extract, and ice cubes.
2. Blend on high speed till the mixture is smooth and creamy. Serve.

Tips: For added sweetness without sugar, consider adding a small amount of stevia or monk fruit extract. You can also add half a peeled cucumber for extra hydration and fiber.

Serving size: One cup

Nutritional values (per serving): Calories: 125; Fat: 3g; Carbs: 7g; Protein: 15g; Sodium: 150mg; Sugar: 0g; Fiber: 2g

8. Ginger Spiced Millet Porridge

Preparation time: Ten mins

Cooking time: Twenty-five mins

Servings: Two

Ingredients:

- One-third cup millet, hulled and rinsed
- Two cups water
- One inch ginger root, peeled and finely grated
- Half tsp cinnamon powder
- One tbsp flaxseed meal
- Two tbsp almonds, slivered and toasted
- Pinch of salt (optional)

Directions:

1. In a medium saucepan, boil two cups of water. Add the rinsed millet along with grated ginger to the boiling water.
2. Cover, then simmer for twenty to twenty-five mins till millet is soft. Stir in cinnamon powder and flaxseed meal till well combined. Cook for additional two mins.
3. Remove, then let it sit covered for five mins. Serve.

Tips: You can top your porridge with fresh berries or sliced banana for natural sweetness. A drizzle of sugar-free almond butter could add richness without added sugars.

Serving size: Half of the total recipe

Nutritional values (per serving): Calories: 220; Fat: 7g; Carbs: 34g; Protein: 6g; Sodium: 40mg; Sugar: 0g; Fiber: 6g

9. Baked Sweet Potato and Egg Boats

Preparation time: Fifteen mins

Cooking time: Thirty mins

Servings: Two

Ingredients:

- One big sweet potato
- Four eggs

- Two tsp olive oil
- One tbsp chopped chives
- One tsp paprika
- One quarter cup shredded reduced-fat cheddar cheese
- Salt & pepper, as required

Directions:

1. Warm up your oven to 400°F. Wash the sweet potato, pat it dry, and pierce it several times with a fork.
2. Place the sweet potato on your baking sheet, drizzle with a tsp of oil, then bake for twenty-five mins or till tender.
3. Cut the sweet potato in half and scoop out the center to create a well, leaving about a half-inch of sweet potato on the skin.
4. Crack an egg into each sweet potato half, sprinkle with paprika, salt, and pepper. Bake for another fifteen mins or till the eggs are set.
5. Drizzle with remaining olive oil, sprinkle with chives and shredded cheese before serving.

Tips: To reduce preparation time, the sweet potatoes can be microwaved for 5-8 mins instead of baking first.

Serving size: One boat

Nutritional values (per serving): Calories: 250; Fat: 10g; Carbs: 20g; Protein: 14g; Sodium: 300mg; Sugar: 5g; Fiber: 3g

10. Flaxseed Meal and Yogurt Parfait

Preparation time: Ten mins

Cooking time: N/A

Servings: One

Ingredients:

- Three quarters cup non-fat Greek yogurt
- Two tbsp flaxseed meal

- One tbsp almond slivers

- Half cup fresh or frozen berries (like strawberries or blueberries)

- One tsp honey (optional)

Directions:

1. In a serving glass, layer half of the Greek yogurt at the bottom. Add one tbsp of flaxseed meal on top of the yogurt layer, then add half of the berries and half of the almond slivers.

2. Repeat layering with the remaining yogurt, flaxseed meal, berries, and almond slivers. Drizzle with honey if desired.

Tips: For added texture add a tbsp of chia seeds to your layers or use toasted almonds for extra crunch.

Serving size: Entire parfait

Nutritional values (per serving): Calories: 280; Fat: 10g; Carbs: 25g; Protein: 20g; Sodium: 85mg; Sugar: 12g (excluding optional honey); Fiber: 8g

11.   Broccoli and Feta Frittata Cups

Preparation time: Ten mins

Cooking time: Twenty-five mins

Servings: Six

Ingredients:

- Two cups of broccoli florets, finely chopped

- Four big eggs

- Quarter cup of feta cheese, crumbled

- One tbsp olive oil

- Quarter tsp of salt

- Quarter tsp of black pepper

- Two tbsp of water

Directions:

1. Warm up your oven to 350°F and lightly oil six muffin cups. Steam the broccoli for three to four mins till just tender, then divide evenly among the muffin cups.

2. In a bowl, whisk eggs, feta cheese, oil, salt, pepper, and water. Pour the egg mixture over the broccoli in the muffin cups.

3. Bake for twenty to twenty-five mins, or till frittata cups are set. Allow cooling for a couple of mins before removing from the muffin tin.

Tips: You can add some fresh herbs like dill or parsley for an additional flavor punch without extra calories.

Serving size: One frittata cup

Nutritional values (per serving): Calories: 110; Fat: 7g; Carbs: 3g; Protein: 9g; Sodium: 210mg; Sugar: 1g; Fiber: 1g

12. Whole-Wheat Banana Pancakes

Preparation time: Ten mins

Cooking time: Fifteen mins

Servings: Four

Ingredients:

- Three-fourths cup of whole-wheat flour
- One ripe banana, mashed
- One big egg
- Half cup low-fat milk
- One tbsp canola oil, plus extra for cooking
- Two tsp baking powder
- Quarter tsp salt

Directions:

1. In your container, mix flour, baking powder, and salt.

2. In another container, beat banana, egg, milk, and canola oil till well blended. Combine it with dry mixture until blended.

3. Heat a non-stick skillet on moderate temp and brush with a little oil. Pour quarter cup measures of batter onto skillet and cook till bubbles form on the surface, then flip and cook till browned.

Tips: Serve with fresh berries or a dollop of yogurt instead of syrup to keep it in line with the fatty liver diet.

Serving size: Two pancakes

Nutritional values (per serving): Calories: 180; Fat: 6g; Carbs: 28g; Protein: 6g; Sodium: 200mg; Sugar: 5g; Fiber: 4g

13.   Sautéed Spinach and Mushrooms on Toast

Preparation time: Five mins

Cooking time: Ten mins

Servings: Two

Ingredients:

- One tbsp olive oil
- Two cups fresh spinach leaves
- One cup sliced mushrooms
- One clove garlic, minced
- One tsp lemon juice
- Two whole-grain toast slices
- Salt & pepper, as required (optional)

Directions:

1. Heat the olive oil in a big pan on moderate temp. Add the minced garlic, then sauté for one minute till fragrant.
2. Adjust to medium-high temp and add the mushrooms, cooking till they begin to soften, approximately three mins.
3. Add the spinach leaves and lemon juice, then cook for two mins till the spinach wilts. Season with salt and pepper if using.

4. Evenly distribute the spinach and mushroom mixture over the toast slices. Serve.

Tips: Use whole grain toast for added fiber content, which is beneficial for a fatty liver diet.

Serving size: One toast topped with half of the sautéed spinach and mushroom mixture

Nutritional values (per serving): Calories: 150; Fat: 7g; Carbs: 18g; Protein: 6g; Sodium: 210mg; Sugar: 2g; Fiber: 5g

14.　　Oatmeal with Sliced Almonds and Blueberries

Preparation time: Five mins

Cooking time: Five mins

Servings: One

Ingredients:

- One cup water or unsweetened almond milk
- Half a cup rolled oats
- Quarter cup blueberries
- One tbsp sliced almonds
- One tsp ground cinnamon
- One tbsp ground flaxseed

Directions:

1. Bring water or almond milk to a boil in your small saucepan. Mix in rolled oats and reduce heat to a simmer.
2. Cook for five mins or till oats are soft. Remove, then mix in ground cinnamon and flaxseed. Pour oatmeal into a serving bowl. Top with blueberries and sliced almonds. Serve.

Tips: Opt for unsweetened almond milk to keep sugar content low and use rolled oats instead of instant oats for better glycemic control which is suitable for people with fatty liver concerns.

Serving size: Entire recipe

Nutritional values (per serving): Calories: 235; Fat: 9g; Carbs: 34g; Protein: 6g; Sodium: 30mg; Sugar: 3g; Fiber: 7g

15.   Egg White Vegetable Scramble

Preparation time: Five mins

Cooking time: Ten mins

Servings: One

Ingredients:

- Four egg whites
- One cup spinach, chopped
- Quarter cup bell peppers, diced
- Two tbsp onion, chopped finely
- One tsp olive oil
- Salt & pepper to taste (optional)

Directions:

1. In a non-stick skillet, heat olive oil on moderate temp. Add onion and bell peppers, then sauté till softened.
2. In your container, beat egg whites till frothy and pour into the skillet with vegetables. Let it sit for a few seconds and then gently scramble with a spatula till fully cooked.
3. Add spinach and cook till wilted. Flavor it with salt and pepper if desired. Serve hot.

Tips: Avoid overcooking the egg whites to keep them tender and moist.

Serving size: Entire recipe

Nutritional values (per serving): Calories 150; Fat 5g; Carbs 6g; Protein 18g; Sodium 170mg; Sugar 3g; Fiber 2g

CHAPTER 3. LUNCH RECIPES

16.   Grilled Chicken Spinach Salad

Preparation time: Fifteen mins

Cooking time: Twenty mins

Servings: Four

Ingredients:

- One lb. boneless skinless chicken breasts
- Four cups fresh spinach leaves
- One cup cherry tomatoes, halved
- Two tbsp olive oil
- One tbsp balsamic vinegar
- One tsp dried oregano
- Quarter tsp salt

Directions:

1. Warm up your grill to medium-high heat. Flavor chicken breasts with salt and dried oregano.
2. Grill chicken for about ten mins on each side or till juices run clear. Let the chicken rest for five mins before slicing.
3. In your big container, toss the spinach with olive oil and balsamic vinegar. Top with cherry tomatoes and grilled chicken slices.

Tips: Use pre-washed spinach to save on preparation time.

Serving size: One-fourth of the total recipe

Nutritional values (per serving): Calories: 230; Fat: 9g; Carbs: 6g; Protein: 30g; Sodium: 220mg; Sugar: 2g; Fiber: 3g

17. Tomato Basil Almond Pesto Pasta

Preparation time: Fifteen mins

Cooking time: Ten mins

Servings: Four

Ingredients:

- One cup fresh basil leaves
- Two tbsp sliced almonds, toasted
- Two cloves garlic
- Three tbsp grated Parmesan cheese
- Quarter cup extra-virgin olive oil
- Eight oz. whole wheat pasta
- One lb. ripe tomatoes, diced

Directions:

1. Cook pasta in your pot with salted-boiling water till tender. Starin, then put aside, reserving one cup of pasta water.
2. Meanwhile, combine basil leaves, toasted almonds, and garlic in your food processor. Pulse till finely chopped.
3. Add Parmesan cheese and continue to process while gradually adding olive oil till a smooth paste forms.
4. Toss the pesto with the drained pasta, adding a bit of reserved pasta water if necessary to loosen the sauce. Gently fold in the diced tomatoes and serve immediately.

Tips: For an extra nutritional boost, substitute regular pasta with high-fiber or legume-based pasta. Keep it light by using less oil and cheese.

Serving size: One & half cups

Nutritional values (per serving): Calories: 350; Fat: 18g; Carbs: 40g; Protein: 10g; Sodium: 160mg; Sugar: 4g; Fiber: 6g

18.   Mediterranean Chickpea Quinoa Bowl

Preparation time: Fifteen mins

Cooking time: Fifteen mins

Servings: Four

Ingredients:

- One cup quinoa, rinsed
- Two cups water
- One (15 oz.) can chickpeas, drained and rinsed
- One big cucumber, diced
- One cup cherry tomatoes, halved
- One tbsp extra-virgin olive oil
- Two tsp lemon juice

Directions:

1. In your medium saucepan, boil quinoa and water. Cover, then simmer for fifteen mins till quinoa is fluffy.
2. In your big container, mix cooked quinoa, chickpeas, cucumber, cherry tomatoes, oil and lemon juice. Flavor it with salt and pepper, then toss to combine well. Serve.

Tips: Add fresh herbs like parsley or mint for an extra flavor punch without additional calories. For added texture, include a spoonful of low-fat feta cheese.

Serving size: Two cups

Nutritional values (per serving): Calories: 330; Fat: 9g; Carbs: 50g; Protein: 14g; Sodium: 200mg; Sugar: 5g; Fiber: 8g

19.   Hearty Vegetable Lentil Soup

Preparation time: Fifteen mins

Cooking time: Thirty-five mins

Servings: Four

Ingredients:

- One cup dry green lentils, washed
- Four cups low-sodium vegetable broth
- One cup diced carrots
- One cup diced celery
- Half a cup diced onion
- Two tbsp tomato paste
- Half tsp dried thyme
- Salt & pepper, as required

Directions:

1. In a big pot, add the lentils and broth, then let it boil. Add carrots, celery, onion, tomato paste, and dried thyme. Flavor it with salt and pepper.
2. Reduce heat, cover, and simmer for thirty mins till lentils are tender. Adjust seasoning if required, and serve hot.

Tips: For extra flavor, sauté the vegetables in olive oil before adding them to the soup. Keep an eye on the broth level and add more if needed during the cooking process.

Serving size: One & half cups

Nutritional values (per serving): Calories: 200; Fat: 1g; Carbs: 36g; Protein: 12g; Sodium: 150mg; Sugar: 4g; Fiber: 15g

20.   Paprika Baked Chicken Thighs

Preparation time: Ten mins

Cooking time: Forty-five mins

Servings: Four

Ingredients:

- Four chicken thighs (approx. one lb.), pat dried
- One tbsp smoked paprika

- One tsp powdered garlic

- Half tsp black pepper

- One tbsp olive oil

Directions:

1. Warm up your oven to 375°F. In a small bowl, combine smoked paprika, powdered garlic, black pepper, and salt if using.

2. Rub olive oil over all sides of the chicken thighs. Apply the spice mixture generously over the chicken thighs.

3. Arrange chicken on a lined baking sheet. Bake for forty-five mins or till the internal temperature reaches 165°F.

Tips: For crispier skin, place the chicken under the broiler for an additional two to three mins at the end of cooking. Let chicken rest for five mins before serving for maximum juiciness.

Serving size: One chicken thigh

Nutritional values (per serving): Calories: 300; Fat: 20g; Carbs: 0g; Protein: 27g; Sodium: 150mg; Sugar: 0g; Fiber: 0g

21. Almond Crusted Trout with Greens

Preparation time: Twenty mins

Cooking time: Fifteen mins

Servings: Four

Ingredients:

- Four (4 oz.) trout fillets

- One cup almond meal

- One tbsp fresh thyme, chopped

- Two tbsp olive oil

- Four cups mixed greens

- One lemon, juiced

- One tsp sea salt

- Half tsp black pepper

Directions:

1. Warm up your oven to 375°F. In a shallow dish, combine almond meal, thyme, sea salt, and black pepper.
2. Coat each trout fillet with the almond mixture and shake off any excess. Heat olive oil in a big ovenproof skillet on moderate-high temp.
3. Add trout fillets to skillet and cook for three to four mins each side till golden brown.
4. Transfer the skillet to the oven and bake for six to seven mins or till fish flakes easily when tested with a fork.
5. Toss mixed greens with lemon juice, and divide them onto plates. Place a baked fillet on top of the greens on each plate.

Tips: Ensure your skillet is hot before adding the fillets to get a nice crust without the fish sticking.

Serving size: One fillet with one cup of greens

Nutritional values (per serving): Calories: 350; Fat: 22g; Carbs: 8g; Protein: 28g; Sodium: 300mg; Sugar: 1g; Fiber: 4g

22. Sautéed Shrimp and Asparagus

Preparation time: Ten mins

Cooking time: Ten mins

Servings: Four

Ingredients:

- One lb. big shrimp, peeled and deveined
- Two cups asparagus, trimmed and cut into one-inch pieces
- One tbsp olive oil
- Three garlic cloves, minced
- One lemon, zest and juice
- Half tsp sea salt

- Quarter tsp black pepper

Directions:

1. Heat olive oil in a big pan on moderate-high temp. Add garlic to the pan and sauté for thirty seconds or till fragrant.
2. Add asparagus to the pan and cook for two mins. Add shrimp to the pan and season with sea salt and black pepper.
3. Cook for five to six mins or till shrimp are pink and cooked through. Remove from heat, add lemon zest and juice; toss well to combine. Serve.

Tips: Don't overcook the shrimp as they can become rubbery if cooked too long. Cut asparagus into even-sized pieces for uniform cooking.

Serving size: Five shrimps with half cup of asparagus

Nutritional values (per serving): Calories: 200; Fat: 6g; Carbs: 5g; Protein: 30g; Sodium: 400mg; Sugar: 2g; Fiber: 2g

23. Spiced Lentil Stew with Kale

Preparation time: Fifteen mins

Cooking time: Thirty mins

Servings: Four

Ingredients:

- Five cups of water
- One cup red lentils, washed
- Two cups kale, chopped
- Half tsp ground cumin
- Half tsp paprika
- One tbsp olive oil
- Salt to taste (minimal)

Directions:

1. In a pot, boil five cups of water, then add red lentils, cumin, paprika, and salt.

2. Adjust to moderate-low temp, then simmer for twenty mins. Add the chopped kale to the lentils and cook for an additional ten mins. Drizzle with olive oil before serving.

Tips: Serve with a slice of whole grain bread for added fiber. Ensure all spices are free from added sugars or additives.

Serving size: One & half cups

Nutritional values (per serving): Calories: 212; Fat: 4g; Carbs: 32g; Protein: 14g; Sodium: 20mg; Sugar: 1g; Fiber: 15g

24. Ginger Soy Poached Cod

Preparation time: Ten mins

Cooking time: Twenty mins

Servings: Four

Ingredients:

- Four (6 oz.) cod fillets
- Four cups of water
- One-inch ginger root, grated
- Two tbsp low-sodium soy sauce
- One tbsp rice vinegar

Directions:

1. In a big skillet or pot, bring water to a slight simmer. Stir in grated ginger root, soy sauce, and rice vinegar.

2. Gently place cod fillets into the poaching liquid. Cook at low heat for twenty mins or till fish flakes easily with a fork.

Tips: Garnish with fresh cilantro for enhanced flavor without added salt. Be cautious not to overcook the cod as it can become dry.

Serving size: One (6 oz.) cod fillet

Nutritional values (per serving): Calories: 189; Fat: 1g; Carbs: 3g; Protein: 40g; Sodium: 330mg; Sugar: 0g; Fiber: 0g

25. Zucchini Ribbon & Chickpea Salad

Preparation time: Fifteen mins

Cooking time: N/A

Servings: Four

Ingredients:

- Two medium zucchinis, sliced into long, thin ribbons
- One cup cooked chickpeas
- One tbsp olive oil
- One tsp fresh lemon juice
- Quarter tsp salt
- One tbsp chopped fresh parsley
- Quarter cup shaved Parmesan cheese

Directions:

1. In your big container, combine the zucchini ribbons with the cooked chickpeas. Drizzle olive oil and lemon juice over the zucchini and chickpeas.
2. Flavor it with salt, add the chopped parsley, and toss gently to combine. Top with shaved Parmesan cheese just before serving.

Tips: For the best texture, use young, firm zucchinis. Ensure your chickpeas are well-drained to avoid excess moisture in the salad.

Serving size: One & half cups

Nutritional values (per serving): Calories: 150; Fat: 7g; Carbs: 16g; Protein: 8g; Sodium: 300mg; Sugar: 3g; Fiber: 5g

26.   Baked Citrus Salmon with Dill

Preparation time: Fifteen mins

Cooking time: Twenty mins

Servings: Four

Ingredients:

- One lb. of fresh salmon fillet
- Two tbsp fresh dill, chopped
- One tsp olive oil
- One tbsp lemon juice
- Half a tsp grated orange zest
- Quarter tsp powdered garlic
- Salt to taste

Directions:

1. Warm up your oven to 400°F. Put salmon fillet on a piece of foil on your baking sheet. Drizzle the olive oil and lemon juice over your salmon.
2. Sprinkle the dill, orange zest, powdered garlic, and salt evenly over the fillet. Wrap the foil around the salmon, sealing it well.
3. Bake for about twenty mins or till the salmon flakes easily with a fork. Serve.

Tips: Ensure your ingredients are fresh for maximum flavor and nutritional value.

Serving size: Quarter lb.

Nutritional values (per serving): Calories: 280; Fat: 15g; Carbs: 1g; Protein: 34g; Sodium: 50mg; Sugar: 0g; Fiber: 0g

27.   Avocado Egg Salad Wraps

Preparation time: Ten mins

Cooking time: N/A

Servings: Two

Ingredients:

- Two hard-boiled eggs, chopped
- Half an avocado, diced
- Half a tbsp of Greek yogurt
- Two big lettuce leaves
- One tsp of Dijon mustard
- One eighth tsp of black pepper
- A pinch of salt

Directions:

1. In your container, mash the avocado and yogurt together till smooth. Mix in chopped eggs, mustard, black pepper, and salt till well combined.
2. Place half of the egg salad mixture onto each lettuce leaf. Roll up the lettuce leaves tightly to enclose the filling.

Tips: You can add some chopped herbs like parsley or chives for extra flavor without adding significant calories or fat.

Serving size: One lettuce wrap filled with half of the egg salad mixture.

Nutritional values (per serving): Calories: 190; Fat: 14g; Carbs: 8g; Protein: 9g; Sodium: 210mg; Sugar: 2g; Fiber: 5g

28.   Quinoa Tofu Buddha Bowl

Preparation time: Twenty-five mins

Cooking time: Twenty mins

Servings: Four

Ingredients:

- Three-fourths cup quinoa, uncooked
- One lb. firm tofu, cubed
- Two cups broccoli florets

- Two cups mixed bell peppers, sliced

- Two tbsp low-sodium soy sauce

- One tbsp sesame oil

- One tsp powdered garlic

Directions:

1. Cook quinoa in your pot with salted-boiling water till tender. Preheat a non-stick pan on moderate temp.

2. Toss tofu cubes with sesame oil and powdered garlic. Sauté tofu for ten mins till golden brown. Steam broccoli florets and bell peppers till tender-crisp.

3. Combine quinoa, vegetables, and tofu in a bowl. Drizzle with low-sodium soy sauce before serving.

Tips: Press the tofu for twenty mins prior to cooking it to remove excess moisture.

Serving size: One-fourth of the total recipe

Nutritional values (per serving): Calories: 320; Fat: 15g; Carbs: 28g; Protein: 22g; Sodium: 470mg; Sugar: 3g; Fiber: 5g

29.   Balsamic Roasted Veggie Platter

Preparation time: Fifteen mins

Cooking time: Twenty-five mins

Servings: Four

Ingredients:

- Two tbsp olive oil

- One tbsp balsamic vinegar

- One tsp dried thyme

- One-quarter tsp of salt

- Two cups broccoli florets

- One cup sliced bell pepper (any color)

- One lb. of baby carrots

Directions:

1. Warm up your oven to 400°F. In your big container, whisk olive oil, balsamic vinegar, thyme, and salt. Add the veggies to the bowl and toss to coat.
2. Spread the vegetables on a baking sheet. Roast for twenty-five mins or till tender and lightly caramelized.

Tips: For variety, try using other vegetables like cauliflower or brussels sprouts.

Serving size: One cup

Nutritional values (per serving): Calories 150; Fat 7g; Carbs 20g; Protein 3g; Sodium 200mg; Sugar 9g; Fiber 5g

30.   Sweet Potato Black Bean Bake

Preparation time: Twenty mins

Cooking time: Thirty-five mins

Servings: Four

Ingredients:

- Three cups sweet potatoes, peeled and diced
- One (15 oz.) can black beans, washed & strained
- One cup corn kernels (fresh or frozen)
- Half tsp of ground cumin
- Half tsp of chili powder
- Two tbsp chopped fresh cilantro
- Four tbsp shredded low-fat cheddar cheese

Directions:

1. Warm up your oven to 375°F. Spread diced sweet potatoes in a baking dish and lightly flavor it with salt and pepper.
2. In your container, mix black beans, corn, cumin, and chili powder. Spread the bean mixture over sweet potatoes. Sprinkle evenly with cheese.

3. Cover with foil and bake for thirty-five mins or till potatoes are soft. Garnish with fresh cilantro before serving.

Tips: Can also be served as a wrap filling or over rice for a more filling meal.

Serving size: One & half cups

Nutritional values (per serving): Calories 320; Fat 5g; Carbs 58g; Protein 12g; Sodium 240mg; Sugar 7g; Fiber 13g

CHAPTER 4. DINNER RECIPES

31. Turmeric Grilled Chicken & Quinoa

Preparation time: Twenty mins

Cooking time: Thirty mins

Servings: Four

Ingredients:

- Four boneless, skinless chicken breasts (about one lb.)
- One cup quinoa, washed
- Two tbsp olive oil
- Two tsp turmeric
- One tsp powdered garlic
- One tsp powdered onion
- Half tsp black pepper
- One & half cups water

Directions:

1. In your small container, mix turmeric, powdered garlic, powdered onion, and black pepper to create a seasoning blend. Rub the seasoning blend onto the chicken breasts evenly.
2. Heat one tbsp of olive oil in a grill pan on moderate temp. Grill chicken for about fifteen mins on each side.
3. In a medium saucepan, boil one and a half cups of water. Add quinoa, adjust to low temp, cover, then simmer for fifteen mins or till all the water is absorbed.
4. Remove the quinoa, then let it stand covered for five mins. Fluff before serving with grilled chicken on top.

Tips: Ensure grill pan is heated properly before adding chicken to prevent sticking.

Serving size: Three-quarters cup of cooked quinoa and one grilled chicken breast

Nutritional values (per serving): Calories 320; Fat 8g; Carbs 27g; Protein 35g; Sodium 95mg; Sugar 1g; Fiber 3g

32.   Mushroom Ragout over Polenta

Preparation time: Ten mins

Cooking time: Twenty mins

Servings: Four

Ingredients:

- One cup polenta
- Three cups water
- One lb. cremini mushrooms, sliced
- One tbsp olive oil
- Two cloves garlic, minced
- One tsp dried thyme
- One half tsp salt
- One fourth cup grated Parmesan cheese (optional for garnish)

Directions:

1. In your medium saucepan, boil water, then gradually stir in the polenta. Reduce the heat to low and cook till the polenta is thick and creamy, stirring occasionally for about fifteen mins.
2. Meanwhile, in a separate pan, heat the olive oil on moderate temp. Add garlic, then sauté for one minute till fragrant.
3. Add mushrooms to the pan with garlic, sprinkle with thyme and salt, and cook till they are soft and browned, about ten mins.
4. Serve the mushroom ragout hot over the cooked polenta. Garnish with Parmesan cheese if desired.

Tips: For a creamier polenta, stir in one tbsp of butter or additional olive oil after it's finished cooking.

Serving size: One cup of cooked polenta with mushroom ragout.

Nutritional values (per serving): Calories 200; Fat 4g; Carbs 37g; Protein 6g; Sodium 300mg; Sugar 2g; Fiber 5g

33.   Turkey and Spinach Stuffed Mushrooms

Preparation time: Fifteen mins

Cooking time: Twenty mins

Servings: Four

Ingredients:

- One cup of spinach, chopped
- Eight oz. ground turkey breast
- Eight big mushrooms, stems removed
- One tbsp olive oil
- Two cloves garlic, minced
- Quarter cup onion, finely chopped
- Half a tsp dried thyme
- Quarter cup of low-fat feta cheese, crumbled

Directions:

1. Warm up your oven to 375°F.
2. In your skillet on moderate temp, sauté the garlic and onions in olive oil till translucent. Add the ground turkey and thyme, cooking till the turkey is no longer pink.
3. Stir in spinach till wilted, remove, then mix in the feta cheese. Stuff each mushroom cap with the turkey mixture.
4. Put them on your baking sheet and bake for fifteen to twenty mins till tender.

Tips: For extra flavor, sprinkle paprika on top before baking. Ensure to choose big mushrooms so they can hold the filling properly.

Serving size: Two stuffed mushrooms

Nutritional values (per serving): Calories: 200; Fat: 9g; Carbs: 8g; Protein: 22g; Sodium: 320mg; Sugar: 3g; Fiber: 2g

34.   Balsamic Glazed Chicken Breast

Preparation time: Ten mins

Cooking time: Twenty-five mins

Servings: Four

Ingredients:

- Four (4 oz.) chicken breasts, boneless and skinless
- One cup balsamic vinegar
- One tbsp raw honey
- Two tbsp olive oil
- Quarter tsp black pepper
- Half tsp sea salt

Directions:

1. In your small saucepan on moderate temp, combine balsamic vinegar and honey. Simmer till reduced by half. Rub chicken breasts with olive oil, salt, and pepper.
2. Grill on moderate-high temp for six to seven mins on each side or till not pink in the center.
3. Once cooked, let rest for five mins before slicing. Serve drizzled with the balsamic reduction.

Tips: Letting the chicken rest after cooking ensures it stays moist when you cut it. For an extra boost of flavor marinate the chicken in some balsamic reduction for thirty mins before grilling.

Serving size: One chicken breast

Nutritional values (per serving): Calories: 210; Fat: 7g; Carbs: 10g; Protein: 28g; Sodium: 380mg; Sugar: 8g; Fiber: 0g

35.   Hearty Eggplant and Chickpea Stew

Preparation time: Fifteen mins

Cooking time: Twenty-five mins

Servings: Four

Ingredients:

- One tbsp olive oil
- Half a cup onions, chopped
- Two cloves garlic, minced
- One medium eggplant, cubed
- One cup canned chickpeas, drained
- Two cups diced tomatoes, no salt added
- One tsp cumin
- One tsp smoked paprika

Directions:

1. Warm up olive oil in a big pot on moderate temp. Add onions and garlic, and sauté till translucent. Add the cubed eggplant and cook for five mins, stirring occasionally.
2. Stir in chickpeas, diced tomatoes, cumin, and smoked paprika. Let it simmer, then cook for twenty mins till the vegetables are tender. Serve.

Tips: Serve with a side of whole grain bread for extra fiber. Garnish with fresh parsley for an additional burst of flavor.

Serving size: One cup

Nutritional values (per serving): Calories 200; Fat 6g; Carbs 30g; Protein 7g; Sodium 300mg; Sugar 9g; Fiber 8g

36. Lightly Blackened Tilapia Filet

Preparation time: Ten mins

Cooking time: Ten mins

Servings: Four

Ingredients:

- Four (one lb.) tilapia filets
- One tbsp olive oil
- One tsp powdered garlic
- One tsp powdered onion
- Half tsp cayenne pepper
- Half tsp dried thyme
- Half tsp black pepper

Directions:

1. Warm up your skillet on moderate-high temp and add the olive oil.
2. Mix powdered garlic, powdered onion, cayenne pepper, dried thyme, and black pepper in your small bowl. Season each filet evenly with the spice mixture.
3. Place filets in the skillet without overcrowding and cook for about four to five mins per side till blackened and fish flakes easily with a fork.

Tips: Keep an eye on the fish to prevent burning due to high heat cooking. Serve with steamed vegetables like broccoli or green beans to keep it liver-friendly.

Serving size: One filet

Nutritional values (per serving): Calories 145; Fat 5g; Carbs 1g; Protein 23g; Sodium 95mg; Sugar 0g; Fiber 0g

37.   Lemon Herb Haddock with Asparagus Spears

Preparation time: Ten mins

Cooking time: Twenty mins

Servings: Four

Ingredients:

- Four (six oz.) haddock fillets
- One lb. fresh asparagus spears, trimmed
- Two tbsp olive oil
- One tsp grated lemon zest
- Two tbsp fresh lemon juice
- One tbsp chopped fresh parsley
- One tsp chopped fresh thyme
- Half tsp sea salt

Directions:

1. Warm up your oven to 400°F. Arrange the haddock fillets in your baking dish.
2. In your container, mix olive oil, zest, lemon juice, parsley, thyme, and sea salt. Brush the fillets with half of the herb mixture.
3. Toss asparagus spears with the remaining herb mixture and arrange around the fish in the dish.
4. Bake for twenty mins or till fish flakes easily and asparagus is tender-crisp. Serve immediately.

Tips: Ensure that your asparagus spears are not too thick; otherwise, they won't cook evenly with the fish. For optimal flavor, use fresh herbs and zest your lemon just before preparing the dish.

Serving size: One haddock fillet with a quarter of the asparagus spears

Nutritional values (per serving): Calories 200; Fat 7g; Carbs 5g; Protein 29g; Sodium 350mg; Sugar 1g; Fiber 2g

38.   Savory Pumpkin and Spinach Curry

Preparation time: Fifteen mins

Cooking time: Thirty mins

Servings: Four

Ingredients:

- Two cups pumpkin cubes
- Four cups fresh spinach leaves
- One cup light coconut milk
- One tbsp olive oil
- One tsp cumin seeds
- Half a tsp turmeric powder
- Three-fourths tsp sea salt

Directions:

1. Warm up oil in a big pan on moderate temp. Add cumin seeds and let them sizzle for about thirty seconds. Add pumpkin cubes to the pan and stir in turmeric powder till well coated.
2. Add coconut milk and sea salt. Cover the pan and let it simmer for about twenty-five mins or till pumpkin is tender.
3. Add spinach leaves to the curry and cook for an additional five mins till spinach is wilted but still vibrant green. Adjust seasoning if necessary and serve hot.

Tips: Pair this curry with quinoa or steamed brown rice for a complete meal that fits within the Fatty Liver Diet guidelines.

Serving size: One cup

Nutritional values (per serving): Calories 125; Fat 5g; Carbs 18g; Protein 3g; Sodium 450mg; Sugar 4g; Fiber 4g

39.   Tofu Kebabs with Tahini Sauce

Preparation time: Fifteen mins

Cooking time: Ten mins

Servings: Four

Ingredients:

- One lb. firm tofu
- Two tbsp olive oil
- One tsp paprika
- Half tsp powdered garlic
- Quarter tsp salt
- One cup bell peppers, cut into pieces

For the Tahini Sauce:

- Two tbsp tahini
- One tbsp lemon juice
- Quarter tsp salt
- Two to four tbsp water (as needed)

Directions:

1. Press the tofu for twenty mins to drain excess water. Cut tofu into cubes.
2. In your container, mix oil, paprika, powdered garlic, and salt. Add tofu and bell peppers, then toss to coat.
3. Thread tofu and peppers alternately onto skewers. Place on a grill pan on moderate temp.
4. Cook for ten mins, turning occasionally till all sides are golden brown.
5. For the tahini sauce, whisk tahini, lemon juice, and salt in a bowl. Gradually add water till desired consistency is reached.
6. Drizzle tahini sauce over the cooked kebabs before serving.

Tips: Pat tofu dry to ensure it gets crispy when cooked. For added flavor marinate the tofu for at least thirty mins.

Serving size: Two kebabs

Nutritional values (per serving): Calories: 250; Fat: 19g; Carbs: 9g; Protein: 19g; Sodium: 320mg; Sugar: 2g; Fiber: 3g

40. Mediterranean Seared Tilapia

Preparation time: Ten mins

Cooking time: Twelve mins

Servings: Four

Ingredients:

- Four tilapia fillets (one lb.)
- Two tbsp olive oil
- Quarter tsp powdered garlic
- Quarter tsp dried oregano
- Quarter tsp salt
- One-eighth tsp black pepper

Directions:

1. Season tilapia fillets with powdered garlic, oregano, salt and black pepper. Warm up oil in your non-stick skillet on moderate-high temp.
2. Add tilapia fillets, then cook for six mins per side or till fish flakes easily. Serve.

Tips: Do not overcrowd the skillet when cooking to ensure the tilapia cooks evenly.

Serving size: One fillet

Nutritional values (per serving): Calories: 200; Fat: 12g; Carbs: 0g; Protein: 23g; Sodium: 170mg; Sugar: 0g; Fiber: 0g

41.   Grilled Tofu with Avocado Salsa

Preparation time: Fifteen mins

Cooking time: Ten mins

Servings: Four

Ingredients:

- One lb. firm tofu
- Two tbsp olive oil
- One tsp powdered garlic
- One big avocado, diced
- One medium tomato, diced
- Two tbsp lime juice
- Quarter cup chopped cilantro
- Salt to taste (optional)

Directions:

1. Press the tofu to remove excess water and cut into half-inch slices. Brush each slice with olive oil and sprinkle with powdered garlic.
2. Grill on moderate temp for five mins on each side or till golden brown.
3. Mix avocado, tomato, lime juice, chopped cilantro, and salt in a bowl to make salsa. Top grilled tofu with the avocado salsa.

Tips: To add extra flavor to your tofu before grilling, let it marinate in a dash of soy sauce or your choice of marinade for thirty mins.

Serving size: One slice of tofu with quarter-cup salsa

Nutritional values (per serving): Calories 190; Fat 14g; Carbs 8g; Protein 12g; Sodium 15mg; Sugar 1g; Fiber 4g

42.   Moroccan Spiced Grilled Veggie Skewers

Preparation time: Twenty mins

Cooking time: Ten mins

Servings: Four

Ingredients:

- Two big bell peppers (any color), cut into one-inch pieces
- One big zucchini, cut into half-inch slices
- Eight cherry tomatoes
- One big red onion, cut into chunks
- Two tbsp olive oil
- One tsp cumin powder
- One tsp paprika

Directions:

1. Warm up your grill to medium-high heat. Thread the bell peppers, zucchini slices, cherry tomatoes, and red onion onto skewers.
2. Brush vegetables with olive oil and evenly sprinkle cumin powder and paprika over them. Grill skewers for ten mins, turning occasionally till veggies are tender and slightly charred.

Tips: Soak wooden skewers in water for thirty mins before using to prevent burning.

Serving size: Two skewers

Nutritional values (per serving): Calories 125; Fat 7g; Carbs 13g; Protein 2g; Sodium 10mg; Sugar 6g; Fiber 3g

43.   Zucchini Noodle Pesto Primavera

Preparation time: Fifteen mins

Cooking time: Ten mins

Servings: Four

Ingredients:

- Two medium zucchinis. spiralized
- One cup cherry tomatoes, halved
- Quarter cup of store-bought or homemade pesto sauce
- One tbsp olive oil
- Half tsp salt
- Quarter tsp black pepper
- Two tbsp of pine nuts (optional)

Directions:

1. In your big pan, heat olive oil on moderate temp. Add the zoodles, sprinkle with salt and pepper, then sauté for about three to five mins till tender.
2. Stir in the cherry tomatoes and cook for an additional two mins. Remove from heat and toss with pesto sauce till the zoodles are well coated. Garnish with pine nuts if using.

Tips: For extra protein, add grilled chicken breast or shrimp to the dish. Do not overcook the zoodles to prevent them from becoming mushy.

Serving size: One-fourth of the recipe

Nutritional values (per serving): Calories: 150; Fat: 12g; Carbs: 8g; Protein: 4g; Sodium: 200mg; Sugar: 4g; Fiber: 3g

44.   Garlic Turkey Meatballs with Tomato Sauce

Preparation time: Twenty mins

Cooking time: Twenty-five mins

Servings: Four

Ingredients:

- One lb. of ground turkey breast
- Two cloves of garlic, minced
- One tbsp fresh thyme leaves

- Half cup of fine almond flour

- One whole egg

- One tsp sea salt

- Half tsp black pepper

For the tomato sauce:

- Two cups of canned crushed tomatoes, no salt added

- One tsp dried oregano

Directions:

1. Warm up your oven to 375°F.

2. In your big container, combine ground turkey, garlic, thyme, almond flour, egg, salt, and pepper.

3. Form mixture into sixteen equal-sized meatballs and place on a lined baking sheet. Bake meatballs for twenty-five mins or till fully cooked through.

4. Meanwhile, pour crushed tomatoes into a saucepan. Add oregano and simmer on low heat till meatballs are ready.

5. Once meatballs are done baking, gently mix them into the tomato sauce.

Tips: Ensure that your canned tomatoes are low sodium or no sodium added options. Serve over additional zucchini noodles for a complete meal.

Serving size: Four meatballs with sauce

Nutritional values (per serving): Calories: 250; Fat: 11g; Carbs: 9g; Protein: 28g; Sodium: 300mg; Sugar: 5g; Fiber: 2g

45. Lemon-Baked Cod with Spinach

Preparation time: Ten mins

Cooking time: Twenty mins

Servings: Four

Ingredients:

- Four cod fillets (about one lb.)
- Four cups fresh spinach leaves
- Two tbsp olive oil
- Two whole lemons (one juiced for two tbsp lemon juice, one sliced)
- Two cloves garlic (minced)
- One half tsp black pepper

Directions:

1. Warm up your oven to 400°F. Place cod fillets in a baking dish coated with one tbsp of olive oil.
2. In your small bowl, combine lemon juice, garlic, and black pepper. Drizzle the mixture over cod fillets. Bake for twelve to fifteen mins or till fish flakes easily.
3. Meanwhile, heat the remaining oil in a big skillet on moderate-high temp. Add spinach leaves and stir frequently till wilted about three to four mins.
4. Serve baked cod on top of wilted spinach and garnish with lemon slices.

Tips: For extra flavor, let cod marinate in lemon juice mixture for thirty mins before baking.

Serving size: One cod fillet with one cup wilted spinach

Nutritional values (per serving): Calories 190; Fat 6g; Carbs 3g; Protein 31g; Sodium 95mg; Sugar 0g; Fiber 1g

CHAPTER 5. SNACK RECIPES

46.   Quinoa Pop Peanut Butter Balls

Preparation time: Fifteen mins

Cooking time: N/A

Servings: Twelve balls

Ingredients:

- One cup puffed quinoa
- Half cup natural peanut butter, unsalted
- Three tbsp honey, preferably raw
- One tsp vanilla extract
- One-fourth tsp ground cinnamon
- Pinch of salt (optional)

Directions:

1. In your big container, combine puffed quinoa, peanut butter, honey, vanilla extract, ground cinnamon, and salt if using. Mix thoroughly till the mixture is well combined.
2. With clean hands or a spoon, take small portions and roll into one-inch balls. Place them on a lined baking sheet.
3. Chill in the refrigerator for at least thirty mins before serving.

Tips: For a firmer texture, you can freeze the balls for about an hour. If your mixture is too dry to form balls, add a bit more peanut butter or honey.

Serving size: One ball

Nutritional values (per serving): Calories: 100; Fat: 6g; Carbs: 9g; Protein: 3g; Sodium: 2mg; Sugar: 4g; Fiber: 1g

47.   **Walnut-Stuffed Prunes**

Preparation time: Ten mins

Cooking time: N/A

Servings: Twelve prunes

Ingredients:

- Twelve pitted prunes
- Twelve walnut halves
- Two tbsp cream cheese, fat-free
- One tbsp orange zest

Directions:

1. Take each prune and carefully open it up at the slit where it was pitted.
2. Stuff each prune with a walnut half and a small dollop of fat-free cream cheese.
3. Sprinkle a pinch of orange zest on top of each stuffed prune.

Tips: For added flavor, you can mix the cream cheese with cinnamon or nutmeg before stuffing. Keep refrigerated till ready to serve to maintain freshness.

Serving size: One stuffed prune

Nutritional values (per serving): Calories: 45; Fat: 2g; Carbs: 7g; Protein: 1g; Sodium: 15mg; Sugar: 4g; Fiber: 1g

48.   **Honey-Drizzled Carrot Chips**

Preparation time: Ten mins

Cooking time: Twenty mins

Servings: Four

Ingredients:

- Two cups thinly sliced carrots
- One tbsp olive oil

- One tbsp honey

- One tsp fresh thyme leaves

- One-fourth tsp salt

- A pinch of black pepper

Directions:

1. Warm up your oven to 375°F. Toss the thinly sliced carrots with oil, thyme, salt, and black pepper in a bowl. Spread the carrots on a baking sheet.

2. Bake for fifteen to twenty mins or till crisp, turning halfway through. Once baked, drizzle honey over the carrot chips while they are still warm.

Tips: Use a mandolin slicer for uniformly thin carrot slices. Watch the chips closely in the last few mins of baking to prevent burning.

Serving size: Half cup of chips

Nutritional values (per serving): Calories: 103; Fat: 3.5g; Carbs: 18g; Protein: 1g; Sodium: 157mg; Sugar: 12g; Fiber: 3g

49. Garlic-Roasted Edamame Snack

Preparation time: Five mins

Cooking time: Fifteen mins

Servings: Four

Ingredients:

- Three cups frozen shelled edamame, washed

- Two cloves garlic, minced

- One tbsp olive oil

- Half a tsp salt

- A quarter tsp black pepper

Directions:

1. Warm up your oven to 400°F. Combine edamame, garlic, oil, salt and pepper in your container.

2. Spread the edamame out in an even layer on a lined baking sheet. Roast for twelve to fifteen mins till golden brown, stirring halfway through.

Tips: Make sure edamame are completely dry after rinsing to ensure they crisp up in the oven.

Serving size: Three-fourths of a cup

Nutritional values (per serving): Calories: 190; Fat: 8g; Carbs: 13g; Protein: 17g; Sodium: 297mg; Sugar: 2g; Fiber: 6g

50.   Almond Butter and Banana Rice Cakes

Preparation time: Five mins

Cooking time: N/A

Servings: Two

Ingredients:

- Two rice cakes
- Two tbsp almond butter
- One banana, sliced
- One tbsp chia seeds

Directions:

1. Spread one tbsp of almond butter evenly over each rice cake.
2. Place half of the banana slices on top of the almond butter on each rice cake.
3. Sprinkle half a tbsp of chia seeds on top of the banana slices for each serving.

Tips: For an extra crunch, toast the rice cakes slightly before adding toppings.

Serving size: One rice cake with toppings

Nutritional values (per serving): Calories 180; Fat 9g; Carbs 23g; Protein 4g; Sodium 45mg; Sugar 7g; Fiber 4g

51.　Spinach and Kale Chips

Preparation time: Ten mins

Cooking time: Twenty mins

Servings: Four

Ingredients:

- Four cups of kale leaves, washed and dried
- Four cups of spinach leaves, washed and dried
- One tbsp olive oil
- One tsp salt
- Half a tsp powdered garlic (optional)

Directions:

1. Warm up your oven to 350°F. In your big container, toss together kale and spinach leaves with olive oil, salt, and powdered garlic till evenly coated.
2. Arrange leaves on a lined baking sheet. Bake for ten to twenty till the edges brown but are not burnt.

Tips: Make sure kale and spinach are thoroughly dried to ensure crispiness.

Serving size: One cup of chips

Nutritional values (per serving): Calories 58; Fat 3.5g; Carbs 6g; Protein 2g; Sodium 240mg; Sugar 0g; Fiber 2g

52.　Cinnamon Sprinkled Baked Pear Slices

Preparation time: Ten mins

Cooking time: Twenty-five mins

Servings: Four

Ingredients:

- Two ripe but firm pears, sliced thinly

- One tbsp ground cinnamon
- One tsp honey (optional)
- Cooking spray (olive oil-based)

Directions:

1. Warm up your oven to 350°F.
2. Arrange the pear slices on a baking sheet coated with cooking spray. Lightly sprinkle cinnamon over the pear slices, and drizzle with honey if desired.
3. Bake for twenty-five mins or till the pears are tender. Remove and allow to cool slightly before serving.

Tips: Choosing pears that are ripe but firm will help them hold their shape when baked.

Serving size: Half a pear sliced

Nutritional values (per serving): Calories: 60; Fat: 0g; Carbs: 16g; Protein: 0g; Sodium: 0mg; Sugar: 12g; Fiber: 3g

53. Fresh Tomato Salsa with Baked Pita Chips

Preparation time: Fifteen mins

Cooking time: Ten mins

Servings: Four

Ingredients:

- Three medium-sized fresh tomatoes, diced
- One tbsp chopped fresh cilantro
- Two tbsp lime juice
- One-fourth tsp salt
- One garlic clove, minced
- Four whole wheat pita bread rounds

Directions:

1. Warm up your oven to 375°F. Combine tomatoes, cilantro, lime juice, salt, and garlic in your container. Let it sit to blend flavors while you prepare the chips.

2. Cut each pita bread into eight triangles and arrange on a baking sheet. Bake for ten mins or till crisp and golden brown. Serve baked pita chips with fresh tomato salsa.

Tips: For a crisper chip, you can lightly spray the pita triangles with cooking spray before baking.

Serving size: Ten chips with salsa

Nutritional values (per serving): Calories: 140; Fat: 1g; Carbs: 29g; Protein: 5g; Sodium: 240mg; Sugar: 4g; Fiber: 4g

54. Herb-Infused Mixed Nuts

Preparation time: Fifteen mins

Cooking time: Ten mins

Servings: Four

Ingredients:

- One cup mixed nuts (almonds, walnuts, pecans)
- One tbsp olive oil
- One tsp dried thyme
- One-half tsp powdered garlic
- One-quarter tsp ground black pepper
- One pinch sea salt (optional)

Directions:

1. Warm up your oven to 350°F.

2. In your container, mix the nuts with olive oil, thyme, powdered garlic, and black pepper till evenly coated.

3. Spread the mixture on a baking sheet, then roast for ten mins or till fragrant. Remove and sprinkle with sea salt if desired.

Tips: You can vary the herbs to include rosemary or oregano for different flavors. Keep an eye on the nuts as they can burn easily due to variations in oven temperatures.

Serving size: Quarter cup

Nutritional values (per serving): Calories: 210; Fat: 20g; Carbs: 6g; Protein: 5g; Sodium: 75mg; Sugar: 1g; Fiber: 3g

55.   Kiwi and Mixed Berries Fruit Salad Bowl

Preparation time: Ten mins

Cooking time: N/A

Servings: Two

Ingredients:

- Two kiwis, peeled and diced
- Half cup blueberries
- Half cup strawberries, hulled and sliced
- Half cup raspberries
- One tbsp fresh mint, chopped
- Two tsp honey (optional)

Directions:

1. In a medium bowl, gently toss diced kiwis, blueberries, strawberries, raspberries, and mint.
2. Drizzle honey over the fruit mixture and toss lightly to combine if you prefer a touch of sweetness.

Tips: The natural sweetness of ripe berries reduces the need for added sugars which is ideal for a fatty liver diet. Chill the fruit salad before serving for a refreshing snack.

Serving size: One cup

Nutritional values (per serving): Calories: 110; Fat: 1g; Carbs: 26g; Protein: 2g; Sodium: 5mg; Sugar: 15g; Fiber: 6g

56.   Cherry Tomato & Mozzarella Skewers

Preparation time: Ten mins

Cooking time: N/A

Servings: Four

Ingredients:

- One cup cherry tomatoes
- One cup mozzarella balls (low-fat)
- Two tbsp extra virgin olive oil
- One tbsp balsamic vinegar
- One tsp dried basil
- Half a tsp salt
- Quarter tsp black pepper

Directions:

1. In your container, whisk oil, balsamic vinegar, basil, salt, and pepper to create the dressing.
2. Thread cherry tomatoes and mozzarella balls alternately on skewers. Drizzle the dressing over the skewers just before serving.

Tips: For added flavor, marinate the mozzarella in the dressing for an hour before assembling.

Serving size: One skewer

Nutritional values (per serving): Calories 150; Fat 9g; Carbs 6g; Protein 8g; Sodium 220mg; Sugar 4g; Fiber 1g

57.   Smoked Salmon & Avocado Nori Rolls

Preparation time: Fifteen mins

Cooking time: N/A

Servings: Two

Ingredients:

- Four sheets nori seaweed
- Half a cup smoked salmon (low sodium)
- One ripe avocado, sliced thinly
- Two tbsp cream cheese (reduced fat)
- One tbsp sesame seeds
- Quarter cup cucumber, cut into matchsticks
- Half a tsp salt

Directions:

1. Lay a sheet of nori on a flat surface. Spread cream cheese thinly over the nori sheet.
2. Place smoked salmon slices, avocado slices, and cucumber matchsticks across the nori sheet. Sprinkle sesame seeds and salt over the filling.
3. Carefully roll up the nori tightly starting from the edge closest to you. Use a sharp knife to cut each roll into bite-sized pieces.

Tips: Wet your knife slightly between cuts to avoid tearing nori sheets.

Serving size: Half of the prepared rolls

Nutritional values (per serving): Calories 220; Fat 9g; Carbs 16g; Protein 12g; Sodium 320mg; Sugar 2g; Fiber 4g

CHAPTER 6. DESSERT RECIPES

58. Coconut Mango Sticky Rice Pudding

Preparation time: Ten mins

Cooking time: Twenty mins

Servings: Four

Ingredients:

- One cup sticky rice (soaked in water for one hour and drained)
- One & quarter cups water
- One cup light coconut milk
- Quarter cup mango, diced
- Two tbsp honey
- One tsp vanilla extract
- Pinch of salt

Directions:

1. In a saucepan, combine the soaked rice and water. Let it boil. Reduce heat to low, cover, and simmer for fifteen to twenty till water is absorbed.
2. Stir in coconut milk, honey, vanilla extract, and a pinch of salt. Cook for another five mins or till pudding thickens.
3. Let it cool slightly and garnish with fresh mango cubes. Serve warm or chilled.

Tips: For added texture, lightly toast the coconut flakes before garnishing.

Serving size: Half a cup

Nutritional values (per serving): Calories 230; Fat 5g; Carbs 40g; Protein 3g; Sodium 30mg; Sugar 6g; Fiber 2g

59. Walnut-Stuffed Poached Pears

Preparation time: Twenty mins

Cooking time: Twenty-five mins

Servings: Four

Ingredients:

- Four ripe pears, peeled, halved, and cored
- One cup water
- Two tbsp lemon juice
- One tsp cinnamon
- Quarter cup chopped walnuts
- One tbsp honey (optional, based on dietary advice)
- One tsp grated ginger

Directions:

1. In a big saucepan on moderate temp, combine water, lemon juice, cinnamon, and ginger.
2. Add pear halves to the saucepan. Cover and simmer for twenty to twenty-five mins or till pears are soft.
3. In a small bowl, mix chopped walnuts with honey if using. Once pears are poached, allow to cool slightly before stuffing with the walnut mixture. Serve warm or chilled.

Tips: Choose firm but ripe pears for the best texture after poaching. You can add a pinch of nutmeg for added flavor if desired.

Serving size: One stuffed pear half

Nutritional values (per serving): Calories: 150; Fat: 5g; Carbs: 27g; Protein: 2g; Sodium: 0mg; Sugar: 17g; Fiber: 6g

60. Cacao Nib Banana Ice Cream

Preparation time: Fifteen mins

Cooking time: N/A

Servings: Four

Ingredients:

- Two ripe bananas, sliced and frozen
- Quarter cup of unsweetened almond milk
- One-third cup of cacao nibs
- One tsp of vanilla extract

Directions:

1. In a food processor, combine the frozen banana slices, almond milk, and vanilla extract. Blend till the mixture is the texture of soft serve ice cream. Stir in cacao nibs by hand.
2. For firmer ice cream, place the mixture into an airtight container and freeze for at least two hours before serving.

Tips: Ensure bananas are ripe and sweet enough to your taste; this dessert relies on the natural sugars from the bananas. If you have difficulty blending, let the bananas thaw slightly before starting the food processor.

Serving size: One cup ice cream

Nutritional values (per serving): Calories: 120; Fat: 5g; Carbs: 20g; Protein: 2g; Sodium: 20mg; Sugar: 10g; Fiber: 3g

61. Coconut Flour Lemon Bars

Preparation time: Twenty mins

Cooking time: Twenty-five mins

Servings: Eight

Ingredients:

- Three big eggs

- One-third cup coconut flour

- One-half cup fresh lemon juice

- Quarter cup honey or a suitable sugar-free sweetener

- Two tbsp unsweetened shredded coconut

- Two tbsp olive oil or melted coconut oil

- One tsp of grated lemon zest

Directions:

1. Warm up your oven to 350°F and grease an 8x8 inch baking dish with oil.

2. In a medium bowl, whisk eggs, lemon juice, honey, and olive oil till well combined. Gradually add in coconut flour till fully incorporated without lumps.

3. Pour batter into prepared baking dish and sprinkle shredded coconut on top. Bake for twenty-five mins or till edges are golden brown and center is set. Allow to cool before cutting into bars.

Tips: Store leftover lemon bars in an airtight container in the refrigerator to maintain freshness. Use parchment paper in the baking dish for easier removal and clean-up.

Serving size: One bar

Nutritional values (per serving): Calories: 130; Fat: 7g; Carbs: 12g; Protein: 3g; Sodium: 40mg; Sugar: 8g; Fiber: 2g

62.   Quinoa Apple Crisp

Preparation time: Twenty mins

Cooking time: Thirty mins

Servings: Four

Ingredients:

- Two cups of cooked quinoa

- Three big apples, peeled and diced

- One tsp of cinnamon

- One tbsp of lemon juice

- Two tbsp of honey

- Quarter cup of walnuts, chopped

- One tsp of coconut oil

Directions:

Warm up your oven to 375°F. Grease an 8x8 inch baking dish with coconut oil.

1. In your big container, mix the cooked quinoa with the diced apples, cinnamon, lemon juice, and honey till all ingredients are well combined.

2. Transfer the quinoa and apple mixture into the baking dish. Evenly sprinkle chopped walnuts on top.

3. Bake for thirty mins or till the top is golden brown and apples are tender. Remove and let it cool slightly before serving.

Tips: Serve warm and if desired, top with a dollop of Greek yogurt for added creaminess.

Serving size: One cup

Nutritional values (per serving): Calories: 235; Fat: 7g; Carbs: 39g; Protein: 5g; Sodium: 10mg; Sugar: 15g; Fiber: 5g

63.　Honey Sweetened Dark Chocolate Bark

Preparation time: Fifteen mins + chilling time

Cooking time: Ten mins

Servings: Six

Ingredients:

- Half a lb. of dark chocolate (at least 70% cacao)

- Quarter cup of slivered almonds

- Two tbsp honey

- One tsp coconut oil

- A pinch of sea salt

- Half a cup of dried cranberries

Directions:

1. Create a double boiler by placing a heatproof bowl over a pot with simmering water, ensuring that the bottom does not touch the water.
2. Break the dark chocolate into pieces and melt in the bowl with coconut oil. Once melted, remove from heat and stir in honey till well combined.
3. Mix in slivered almonds and dried cranberries.
4. Pour chocolate mixture onto a parchment-lined baking tray and spread out evenly with a spatula.
5. Sprinkle sea salt over the chocolate mixture. Refrigerate for at least two hours or till firm. Break into pieces before serving.

Tips: Store any leftovers in an airtight container in the refrigerator to keep the bark crisp.

Serving size: One oz.

Nutritional values (per serving): Calories: 219; Fat: 14g; Carbs: 23g; Protein: 3g; Sodium: 20mg; Sugar: 18g; Fiber: 3g

64. Pumpkin Spiced Baked Yogurt

Preparation time: Ten mins

Cooking time: Twenty-five mins

Servings: Four

Ingredients:

- One cup plain Greek yogurt
- Quarter cup pumpkin puree (not pie filling)
- Two tbsp maple syrup
- One-half tsp pumpkin pie spice
- One tsp vanilla extract

Directions:

1. Warm up your oven to 350°F.

2. In your container, mix yogurt, pumpkin puree, maple syrup, pumpkin pie spice, and vanilla extract. Divide the mixture among four oven-safe ramekins.

3. Put ramekins in your baking dish and fill the dish with boiling water halfway up the sides of the ramekins.

4. Bake for twenty-five mins, or till the yogurt is set but still jiggly in the center.

Tips: Top with a sprinkle of chopped nuts or a drizzle of extra maple syrup if desired. Can be served warm or chilled.

Serving size: One ramekin

Nutritional values (per serving): Calories 120; Fat 2g; Carbs 14g; Protein 8g; Sodium 45mg; Sugar 11g; Fiber 0.5g

65. Maple Glazed Grilled Peaches

Preparation time: Ten mins

Cooking time: Ten mins

Servings: Four

Ingredients:

- Four medium peaches, halved and pitted
- Two tbsp pure maple syrup
- One-half tsp ground cinnamon
- One tbsp unsalted butter, melted
- Fresh mint for garnish (optional)

Directions:

1. Warm up your grill to medium-high heat.

2. In your small container, mix maple syrup, cinnamon, and melted butter. Brush the cut sides of the peaches with the maple mixture.

3. Put peaches cut side down on your grill and cook for five mins till grill marks appear.

4. Flip over and brush with more of the maple mixture. Grill for another three to five mins till peaches are tender and caramelized.

Tips: Serve with a dollop of Greek yogurt or low-fat ice cream if desired. Can also be made by broiling in an oven if a grill is not available.

Serving size: Two peach halves

Nutritional values (per serving): Calories 110; Fat 2g; Carbs 22g; Protein 1g; Sodium 0mg; Sugar 20g; Fiber 3g

66.   Citrus Berry Salad with Honey Mint Dressing

Preparation time: Ten mins

Cooking time: N/A

Servings: Four

Ingredients:

- Two cups mixed berries (strawberries, blueberries, raspberries)
- One big orange, peeled and segmented
- One tbsp fresh mint leaves, finely chopped
- Two tbsp honey
- One tsp fresh lemon juice

Directions:

1. In your big container, mix berries and orange segments.
2. In your small container, whisk honey, lemon juice, and mint leaves till well blended.
3. Drizzle the honey mint dressing over the berry mixture and gently toss to coat. Refrigerate for five mins to allow flavors to meld.

Tips: For the best flavor, use fresh berries and organic honey. The salad can also be enjoyed as a refreshing snack any time of the day.

Serving size: One cup

Nutritional values (per serving): Calories 90; Fat 0g; Carbs 22g; Protein 1g; Sodium 5mg; Sugar 16g; Fiber 4g

67.   Date and Nut Energy Balls

Preparation time: Fifteen mins

Cooking time: N/A

Servings: Eight

Ingredients:

- One cup pitted dates
- Half cup raw almonds
- Quarter cup shredded coconut (unsweetened)
- One tbsp chia seeds
- One tbsp flax seeds
- Half tsp ground cinnamon
- Quarter tsp sea salt

Directions:

1. Add dates to a food processor and pulse till they form a sticky dough-like consistency.
2. Add almonds, coconut, chia seeds, flax seeds, cinnamon, and salt. Pulse till well combined and mixture sticks together.
3. Using your hands, roll the mixture into balls, then keep them in the refrigerator till ready to serve.

Tips: If the date mixture is too dry to form balls, add a tbsp of water to help it stick together. Feel free to roll energy balls in extra shredded coconut or chopped nuts for added texture.

Serving size: One energy ball

Nutritional values (per serving): Calories 120; Fat 7g; Carbs 16g; Protein 2g; Sodium 75mg; Sugar 12g; Fiber 3g

68.   Fresh Fig with Ricotta and Pistachios

Preparation time: Five mins

Cooking time: N/A

Servings: Four

Ingredients:

- Eight fresh figs, halved
- One-half cup ricotta cheese
- Quarter cup pistachios, roughly chopped
- Two tbsp honey
- Pinch of cinnamon (optional)

Directions:

1. Arrange halved figs on a serving platter. Spoon the ricotta cheese evenly over the fig halves.
2. Drizzle honey over the cheese and figs. Sprinkle chopped pistachios and a pinch of cinnamon if desired.

Tips: Choose ripe but firm figs for best results.

Serving size: Two fig halves with topping

Nutritional values (per serving): Calories 150; Fat 7g; Carbs 21g; Protein 5g; Sodium 45mg; Sugar 16g; Fiber 3g

CHAPTER 7. DRINKS AND BEVERAGES

69.   Dandelion Detox Tea

Preparation time: Five mins

Cooking time: Ten mins

Servings: Two servings

Ingredients:

- One tbsp of dried dandelion leaves
- Two cups of boiling water
- One tsp of honey (optional)
- One tsp of lemon juice (fresh)

Directions:

1. Put dried dandelion leaves into a teapot or heatproof pitcher. Pour the boiling water over the leaves and let steep for ten mins.
2. Strain the tea into cups and add honey (if using) and fresh lemon juice to taste.

Tips: For best results, use organic dandelion leaves to ensure there are no added chemicals or pesticides. You can also add mint leaves for a refreshing twist.

Serving size: One cup

Nutritional values (per serving): Calories 2; Fat 0g; Carbs 0.5g; Protein 0g; Sodium 2mg; Sugar 0g; Fiber 0g

70.   Berry Citrus Hydration Infused-Water

Preparation time: Five mins

Cooking time: N/A

Servings: Four

Ingredients:

- One cup of mixed fresh berries (strawberries, blueberries, raspberries)
- One tbsp of fresh mint leaves
- One medium lemon, thinly sliced
- Four cups of ice-cold water

Directions:

1. In a big pitcher, gently muddle the mixed fresh berries and mint leaves. Add the thin slices of lemon to the pitcher.
2. Pour ice-cold water over the fruit mixture. Cover the pitcher and refrigerate for at least one hour or overnight to infuse flavors. Stir well before serving.

Tips: Use a wooden spoon or a muddler to muddle the fruits gently; do not pulverize the fruits. You can prepare this water in advance and keep it refrigerated for up to three days for best flavor.

Serving size: One cup

Nutritional values (per serving): Calories 18; Fat 0g; Carbs 4.8g; Protein 0.3g; Sodium 7mg; Sugar 3.1g; Fiber 1.2g

71. Lemon Lavender Healing Water

Preparation time: Five mins

Cooking time: N/A

Servings: Four

Ingredients:

- Four cups of ice-cold water
- One medium lemon, thinly sliced
- Two tsp of dried lavender buds

Directions:

1. Place thinly sliced lemons in a big pitcher. Sprinkle dried lavender buds over the lemon slices. Fill the pitcher with ice-cold water.
2. Cover and let it refrigerate overnight or at least four hours to allow the lavender and lemon to infuse into the water. Strain out lavender buds before serving.

Tips: Using dried lavender buds suitable for culinary uses ensures that they are free from pesticides and additives. If you find the lavender flavor too strong, reduce infusion time accordingly.

Serving size: One cup

Nutritional values (per serving): Calories 6; Fat 0g; Carbs 2g; Protein 0.1g; Sodium 0mg; Sugar 0.6g; Fiber 0.3g

72. Lemon Ginger Soothe Tea

Preparation time: Five mins

Cooking time: Ten mins

Servings: Two

Ingredients:

- One tbsp fresh ginger root, peeled and thinly sliced
- Two cups of water
- One tbsp lemon juice, freshly squeezed
- One tsp honey (optional and to taste)

Directions:

1. In a medium saucepan, bring two cups of water to a boil. Add the sliced ginger to the boiling water and let it simmer for ten mins.
2. Remove from heat and strain the tea into cups. Add the freshly squeezed lemon juice to each cup. Sweeten with honey to taste if desired, stirring till dissolved.

Tips: For an extra anti-inflammatory boost, add a pinch of ground turmeric to the boiling water with ginger.

Serving size: One cup

Nutritional values (per serving): Calories: 24; Fat: 0g; Carbs: 6g; Protein: 0g; Sodium: 1mg; Sugar: 1g (without honey); Fiber: 0g

73.   Cucumber Mint Refresh Water

Preparation time: Five mins

Cooking time: N/A

Servings: Four

Ingredients:

- One medium cucumber, thinly sliced
- Four cups of cold filtered water
- Four tbsp fresh mint leaves, loosely packed
- Ice cubes (optional)

Directions:

1. In a big pitcher, combine the sliced cucumber and fresh mint leaves. Add four cups of cold filtered water.
2. Stir gently and refrigerate for at least one hour or overnight for intensified flavors. Serve chilled with ice cubes if desired.

Tips: To keep your Refresh Water flavorful without dilution as ice melts, freeze some cucumber slices in ice cube trays filled with water and add these cubes to your drink instead of regular ice cubes.

Serving size: One cup

Nutritional values (per serving): Calories: Less than Five; Fat: 0g; Carbs: 1g; Protein: 0g; Sodium: 2mg; Sugar: 0g; Fiber: 0g

74.   Silymarin Milk Thistle Brew

Preparation time: Five mins

Cooking time: Fifteen mins

Servings: Two

Ingredients:

- One tbsp of milk thistle seeds, crushed
- Two cups of water
- One tsp of honey (optional)

Directions:

1. Crush the milk thistle seeds gently with a mortar and pestle. Bring water to a boil in a small saucepan, then add the crushed seeds.
2. Reduce heat and simmer for fifteen mins. Remove from heat and strain into cups, add honey if desired.

Tips: Crushing the milk thistle seeds before brewing helps to release silymarin, which is beneficial for liver health. Drink this brew on an empty stomach for better absorption.

Serving size: One cup

Nutritional values (per serving): Calories 9; Fat 0g; Carbs 2g; Protein 0g; Sodium 12mg; Sugar 1g (adds calories if honey is used); Fiber 0g

75. Celery Apple Purify Juice

Preparation time: Five mins

Cooking time: N/A

Servings: Two

Ingredients:

- One & half cups of water
- Four stalks of celery
- Two big apples, cored and sliced
- One tbsp of fresh lemon juice
- One tsp of grated ginger
- A handful of fresh parsley leaves (optional)

Directions:

1. Wash the celery and apples thoroughly. Chop the celery into smaller pieces if necessary to fit your juicer.
2. Process the celery, apples, lemon juice, ginger, and parsley (if using) through a juicer. Stir the juice well before pouring into glasses. Serve.

Tips: For added benefits, you can include a pinch of turmeric or sprinkle of chia seeds before serving.

Serving size: 1 glass

Nutritional values (per serving): Calories 95; Fat 0.2g; Carbs 24g; Protein 1g; Sodium 32mg; Sugar 18g; Fiber 4.5g

76.   Kale Pineapple Rejuvenation Smoothie

Preparation time: Ten mins

Cooking time: N/A

Servings: Two

Ingredients:

- Two cups of chopped kale leaves, stems removed
- One cup of frozen pineapple chunks
- One medium banana, sliced
- Three-quarters cup of unsweetened almond milk
- Half tbsp of chia seeds
- Half tsp of freshly squeezed lemon juice

Directions:

1. Place the kale, pineapple, banana, almond milk, chia seeds, and lemon juice in a blender.
2. Blend on high speed till smooth and creamy. Pour the smoothie into two glasses and serve immediately.

Tips: If you prefer a colder smoothie, you can freeze the banana slices before adding them to the blender.

Serving size: 1 glass

Nutritional values (per serving): Calories 145; Fat 2g; Carbs 30g; Protein 4g; Sodium 56mg; Sugar 16g; Fiber 5g

77. Papaya Digestive Boost Smoothie

Preparation time: Five mins

Cooking time: N/A

Servings: Two

Ingredients:

- One & half cups diced papaya
- One cup unsweetened almond milk
- One tbsp chia seeds
- Half a tsp ground ginger
- Half a tsp cinnamon powder
- Ice cubes (optional)

Directions:

1. Combine the papaya, almond milk, chia seeds, ground ginger, and cinnamon in a blender. Blend on high speed till smooth.
2. Add ice cubes if desired and blend till your preferred consistency is reached.

Tips: For an extra protein boost, add one scoop of plant-based protein powder.

Serving size: One cup

Nutritional values (per serving): Calories 150; Fat 3g; Carbs 24g; Protein 3g; Sodium 96mg; Sugar 13g; Fiber 5g

78.   Almond Milk Green Goddess Smoothie

Preparation time: Five mins

Cooking time: N/A

Servings: Two

Ingredients:

- Two cups fresh spinach leaves
- One cup unsweetened almond milk
- Half a ripe avocado
- One tbsp fresh lemon juice
- One tbsp flaxseed meal
- Four ice cubes

Directions:

1. Place the spinach, almond milk, avocado, lemon juice, and flaxseed meal in a blender.
2. Add ice cubes to the blender. Blend on high speed till the mixture is smooth.

Tips: If you prefer a sweeter taste, add a few drops of stevia. Ensure that your avocado is ripe for creaminess.

Serving size: One cup

Nutritional values (per serving): Calories 114; Fat 9g; Carbs 8g; Protein 2g; Sodium 50mg; Sugar Less than 1g; Fiber 4g

79.   Carrot Turmeric Anti-Inflammatory Juice

Preparation time: Ten mins

Cooking time: N/A

Servings: Two

Ingredients:

- Four big carrots

- One inch of fresh turmeric root

- Half a lemon, peeled

- One tbsp of flaxseed oil

- One tsp of honey (optional)

- One fourth tsp of ground black pepper

- Two cups of cold water

Directions:

1. Wash and peel the carrots and turmeric root. Cut the carrots into manageable pieces for your juicer.

2. Add the carrots, turmeric, and peeled lemon through the juicer. Stir in flaxseed oil, honey if using it for taste, and black pepper.

3. Pour the juice over ice in two glasses or blend with cold water to dilute to your preference.

Tips: Drink immediately to get the benefits of all nutrients. If you don't have fresh turmeric root, you can substitute with half a tsp of ground turmeric.

Serving size: One cup

Nutritional values (per serving): Calories: 152; Fat: 7g; Carbs: 21g; Protein: 2g; Sodium: 76mg; Sugar: 9g; Fiber: 6g

80. Beetroot and Ginger Liver Support Juice

Preparation time: Ten mins

Cooking time: N/A

Servings: Two

Ingredients:

- Three medium-sized beetroots

- One apple

- One inch of ginger root

- Half a lemon, peeled

- One tbsp of olive oil

- Two cups of cold water

Directions:

1. Scrub the beetroots and ginger root thoroughly and peel them if they are not organic. Core the apple and cut it along with the beetroots into pieces that will fit your juicer.

2. Push the beetroot pieces, apple, ginger, and peeled lemon through your juicer. Add olive oil to the extracted juice and stir well.

3. Serve the juice immediately over ice or mixed with cold water according to taste preference.

Tips: For added health benefits include a pinch of cayenne pepper. Drinking beet juice may color your urine red which is harmless.

Serving size: One cup

Nutritional values (per serving): Calories: 135; Fat: 7g; Carbs: 18g; Protein: 2g; Sodium: 65mg; Sugar: 13g; Fiber: 4g

CONCLUSION

As we close the final pages of the ***"Fatty Liver Diet Cookbook,"*** it's vital to recognize that embarking on a journey to reverse fatty liver disease is about more than following recipes; it's about embracing a lifestyle change that values nutrition, understands the importance of exercise, and prioritizes your overall well-being. Throughout this book, we've explored various aspects of managing a fatty liver through diet. We delved into the types of foods that support liver health, those we should limit or avoid, and how to make sense of nutrition labels.

The recipes curated from breakfast to dinner are not just meals; they are stepping stones on the path to a healthier liver and body. Breakfast options like the *Avocado and Spinach Smoothie Bowl* kick-start your metabolism with wholesome ingredients. Lunches such as the *Mediterranean Chickpea Quinoa Bowl* ensure midday sustenance without compromising on flavor or nutrition. Dinners, like the *Turmeric Grilled Chicken & Quinoa*, provide hearty nourishment while aligning with the diet's principles.

We didn't stop at solid meals; snacks like *Walnut-Stuffed Prunes* and *Kiwi Mixed Berries Fruit Salad Bowl*, desserts such as *Coconut Mango Sticky Rice Pudding* and *Maple Glazed Grilled Peaches*, and a variety of drinks ranging from *Dandelion Detox Tea* to *Kale Pineapple Rejuvenation Smoothie* were included to offer full-range options for every craving and time of day.

But remember, recipes alone won't cure a fatty liver. Incorporating lifestyle changes such as regular exercise, stress reduction techniques, better sleep hygiene, and staying motivated with help from support groups is crucial for success. Setbacks are normal; what's important is getting back on track with perseverance and dedicated effort.

For anyone feeling overwhelmed by all this information, here's one final piece of advice: start small. Choose one meal from each chapter you feel excited to try; focus on incorporating one new healthy habit at a time. Perhaps begin with preparing your lunch ahead or joining a local walking group. Each small step supports your larger goal.

We hope this cookbook serves not just as a collection of recipes but as an educational guide and motivational resource. As you transition into this new way of eating and living, allow yourself patience and grace—the journey towards healing takes time but is immensely rewarding. Here's to your health and happiness—may every bite you take be one step closer to a healthier liver and life.

28-DAY MEAL PLAN

DAY	BREAKFAST	LUNCH	DINNER	SNACK/DESSERT
1	Avocado and Spinach Smoothie Bowl	Grilled Chicken Spinach Salad	Turmeric Grilled Chicken & Quinoa	Quinoa Pop Peanut Butter Balls
2	Egg White Vegetable Scramble	Sweet Potato Black Bean Bake	Lemon-Baked Cod with Spinach	Coconut Mango Sticky Rice Pudding
3	Oatmeal with Sliced Almonds and Blueberries	Balsamic Roasted Veggie Platter	Garlic Turkey Meatballs with Tomato Sauce	Smoked Salmon & Avocado Nori Rolls
4	Sautéed Spinach and Mushrooms on Toast	Quinoa Tofu Buddha Bowl	Zucchini Noodle Pesto Primavera	Fresh Fig with Ricotta and Pistachios
5	Low-Fat Greek Yogurt with Nuts and Honey	Avocado Egg Salad Wraps	Moroccan Spiced Grilled Veggie Skewers	Cherry Tomato & Mozzarella Skewers
6	Whole-Wheat Banana Pancakes	Sautéed Shrimp and Asparagus	Lemon Herb Haddock with Asparagus Spears	Date and Nut Energy Balls
7	Broccoli and Feta Frittata Cups	Baked Citrus Salmon with Dill	Grilled Tofu with Avocado Salsa	Kiwi and Mixed Berries Fruit Salad Bowl
8	Flaxseed Meal and Yogurt Parfait	Zucchini Ribbon & Chickpea Salad	Mediterranean Seared Tilapia	Citrus Berry Salad with Honey Mint Dressing
9	Baked Sweet Potato and Egg Boats	Spiced Lentil Stew with Kale	Tofu Kebabs with Tahini Sauce	Almond Butter and Banana Rice Cakes
10	Sugar-Free Spirulina Protein Shake	Ginger Soy Poached Cod	Savory Pumpkin and Spinach Curry	Maple Glazed Grilled Peaches

11	Ginger Spiced Millet Porridge	Tomato Basil Almond Pesto Pasta	Mushroom Ragout over Polenta	Herb-Infused Mixed Nuts
12	Kale and Turkey Breakfast Hash	Almond Crusted Trout with Greens	Lightly Blackened Tilapia Filet	Walnut-Stuffed Poached Pears
13	Tofu Scramble with Mixed Peppers	Paprika Baked Chicken Thighs	Hearty Eggplant and Chickpea Stew	Fresh Tomato Salsa with Baked Pita Chips
14	Herbed Chicken Sausage Patties	Mediterranean Chickpea Quinoa Bowl	Turkey and Spinach Stuffed Mushrooms	Pumpkin Spiced Baked Yogurt
15	Chia Seed and Almond Pudding	Hearty Vegetable Lentil Soup	Balsamic Glazed Chicken Breast	Spinach and Kale Chips
16	Avocado and Spinach Smoothie Bowl	Grilled Chicken Spinach Salad	Turmeric Grilled Chicken & Quinoa	Honey Sweetened Dark Chocolate Bark
17	Egg White Vegetable Scramble	Sweet Potato Black Bean Bake	Lemon-Baked Cod with Spinach	Cinnamon Sprinkled Baked Pear Slices
18	Oatmeal with Sliced Almonds and Blueberries	Balsamic Roasted Veggie Platter	Garlic Turkey Meatballs with Tomato Sauce	Quinoa Apple Crisp
19	Sautéed Spinach and Mushrooms on Toast	Quinoa Tofu Buddha Bowl	Zucchini Noodle Pesto Primavera	Walnut-Stuffed Prunes
20	Low-Fat Greek Yogurt with Nuts and Honey	Avocado Egg Salad Wraps	Moroccan Spiced Grilled Veggie Skewers	Cacao Nib Banana Ice Cream
21	Whole-Wheat Banana Pancakes	Sautéed Shrimp and Asparagus	Lemon Herb Haddock with Asparagus Spears	Garlic-Roasted Edamame Snack
22	Broccoli and Feta Frittata Cups	Baked Citrus Salmon with Dill	Grilled Tofu with Avocado Salsa	Coconut Flour Lemon Bars
23	Flaxseed Meal and Yogurt Parfait	Zucchini Ribbon & Chickpea Salad	Mediterranean Seared Tilapia	Honey-Drizzled Carrot Chips

24	Baked Sweet Potato and Egg Boats	Spiced Lentil Stew with Kale	Tofu Kebabs with Tahini Sauce	Quinoa Pop Peanut Butter Balls
25	Sugar-Free Spirulina Protein Shake	Ginger Soy Poached Cod	Savory Pumpkin and Spinach Curry	Coconut Mango Sticky Rice Pudding
26	Ginger Spiced Millet Porridge	Tomato Basil Almond Pesto Pasta	Mushroom Ragout over Polenta	Smoked Salmon & Avocado Nori Rolls
27	Kale and Turkey Breakfast Hash	Almond Crusted Trout with Greens	Lightly Blackened Tilapia Filet	Fresh Fig with Ricotta and Pistachios
28	Tofu Scramble with Mixed Peppers	Paprika Baked Chicken Thighs	Hearty Eggplant and Chickpea Stew	Cherry Tomato & Mozzarella Skewers

MEASUREMENTS AND CONVERSIONS

VOLUME EQUIVALENTS (LIQUID)		
US STANDARD	**US OUNCES**	**METRIC (APPROX.)**
1 tsp	1/6 oz	5 ml
1 tbsp	1/2 oz	15 ml
1 fluid ounce	1 oz	30 ml
1 cup	8 oz	240 ml
1 pint	16 oz	475 ml
1 quart	32 oz	950 ml
1 gallon	128 oz	3.8 L

VOLUME EQUIVALENTS (DRY)		WEIGHT EQUIVALENTS	
US STANDARD	**METRIC (APPROX.)**	**US STANDARD**	**METRIC (APPROX.)**
1/4 tsp	1.25 ml	1 ounce	28 g
1/2 tsp	2.5 ml	4 ounces	113 g
1 tsp	5 ml	8 ounces	225 g
1/4 cup	60 ml	12 ounces	340 g
1/3 cup	80 ml	One pound (16oz)	455 g
1/2 cup	120 ml		
1 cup	240 ml		

<h1 style="text-align:center">OVEN TEMPERATURES</h1>

FAHRENHEIT	CELSIUS (APPROX.)
200° F	93° C
225° F	107° C
250° F	121° C
275° F	135° C
300° F	149° C
325° F	163° C
350° F	177° C
375°F	191° C
400°F	204° C
425°F	218°C

Note: The values in the tables are approximate and should be used for reference as a guide when cooking.